DEDICATION

*I dedicate this book to my ER folks.
First, to my beloved ER nurses: There's nobody like you.
Your selflessness, your dedication to your patients, your courage, your loyalty, and your humor put you in a class of your own. I am honored to have worked with every one of you.
You always had my back in the ER. You also stood by me when my writing got hijacked and my soul stolen.
Thank you. I wish I had better words.
Gina Garbino, I'm lucky to have you as a friend. Years later, I still don't know what happened that day Vicky disappeared. But you held down the fort, and nobody died. I'm so proud of you and your impressive career!
Emmalee Colby, thank you for always having my back. From standing up for me when your patients got upset that I kept asking you the hard questions to helping my patients even when they weren't yours, every shift was better with you there. I'm proud of everything you have accomplished, and I wish I were half the mom you are.
Laurie Fregeau Clark, thank you for many years of friendship and your trust and support. I'm amazed at the success story you have become. You've built yourself*

into this beautiful, strong, and healthy woman. I'm glad that I got to watch you.

Kim Branham, thank you for your support. You are kind but also such a fighter. Thank you for helping me through one of my hardest spots. Who knew writing was easy and refraining from strangling people afterward was hard?

Tiffany Kirk, thank you for standing up for me. I wish we got to spend more time together. Every shift working with you was a joy. You're bright, funny, and kind. You are a fantastic patient advocate. I always knew my patients were safe with you.

Jess Sovie, thank you for your friendship and loyalty. Your tremendous energy, sense of humor, and brilliance made every time I worked with you a joy. I am so lucky to have worked with you, and I love watching you soar.

Natalie Rachel, thank you for fighting for me. I hope we get to compare notes on writing someday.

Thanks to all of you, too many to name - this book is too short for you all. I'm humbled and grateful for your friendship, loyalty, and kindness. I hope I did something somewhere to deserve it. If I didn't, I hope I do someday.

This book is not mine. It's ours. It's the closest I could come to putting our strange ER life into words. It's about our work, struggles, and endless daily fights. Every shift, we fight death, we fight the EHR, we fight time, we fight Darwin, we fight the administration and many other things that I can't remember right now. The one thing I know is that we're all in this together.

My life, work, and I are better because of you.

Thank you.

Love you all.

Rada

STAY AWAY FROM MY ER AND OTHER FUN BITS OF WISDOM

WOBBLING BETWEEN HUMOR AND HEARTBREAK

RADA JONES MD

APOLODOR

The names of individuals and places have been changed to maintain their anonymity. Identifying characteristics and details such as age, gender, physical properties and occupations have also been changed to protect privacy.

Copyright © 2020 by Rada Jones MD

All rights reserved.

No part of this book may be reproduced in any form or by any electronic or mechanical means, including information storage and retrieval systems, without written permission from the author, except for the use of brief quotations in a book review.

FOREWORD

Dear Reader,

If you're sensitive and easily offended, don't bother with this book. Like the ER, this book is gritty, coarse, and full of gallows humor. We laugh at things most people don't. That stops us from crying and allows us to return to the job day after terrible day.

As Katherine Watson, a medical ethicist from Northwestern University's Feinberg School of Medicine, said: "the butt of the doctors' humor is not the patient. It's death." Humor helps us "integrate this terrible event and get through the shift," and move on to caring for the next patient.

"Stay Away from my ER, and other fun bits of wisdom" is a collection of ~~rants~~ essays that I wrote while practicing medicine. I used my words to depict what ER life is like: The doubt, the frustration, the adrenaline rush, the despair, the camaraderie, the pain, the dark humor, the losses.

Some are funny.

Some are not funny at all. They're sad, tragic even, since life in the ER is the farthest thing from comedy. In the ER, people die every day, or lose things that are more precious to them than their lives.

Some of my essays ask questions I can't answer. What is and what isn't ethical about organ transplants? What should we do about the disappearance of Emergency Nurses? How can we improve mental health care?

Some essays tackle the thorny issue of American healthcare. We may or may not agree on the solutions, but I hope we can agree that our healthcare needs to improve.

There's one thing all my essays have in common: they are all true. They are the absolute, raw, unadulterated truth. Everything I wrote about happened - again and again. The fight with the EMRs, shampoo bottles lodging where they don't belong, women coming to get checked for prostate cancer after googling their symptoms - it all happened. Again and again.

I hope this book will be fun and will teach you about the ER. If neither happens, then I didn't do my job.

Thank you for reading me.
Rada

CONTENTS

Stay Away From My ER: A few tips	1
The Hemorrhage of Emergency Nurses	7
The ER Laws	13
Death by Patient Satisfaction	17
I'm an ER Doc and I Have No Friends	23
Strangest Real Patient Complaints, Part 1	27
Put Me to Sleep	31
13 Reasons to Choose a Woman Doctor	35
VOMIT: Victims of Modern Information Technology	39
Recycle Thyself	45
Why I Never Tell People I'm a Doctor	53
Healthcare Costs and the Provider Curse	57
Strangest Real Patient Complaints, Part 2	63
Sex and the Silver Foxes	67
40 Pro Tips for Your Loved One's ER Visit	71
Crazy!	79
Twenty-four Reasons to NOT Vaccinate Your Kid	85
Why Doctors Make Bad Patients	91
What's So Hard About the ER?	97
Strangest Real Patient Complaints, Part 3	103
Obamacare vs. Universal Healthcare	107
Patients Say the Darnedest Things	113
The Pill	123
Stay Away From My ER: More Tips	129
The Perfect Doctor	133
More ER Laws	137

Do You Speak ER?	143
Lessons from My Patients	149
About the Author	153
Overdose: An Excerpt	157

STAY AWAY FROM MY ER: A FEW TIPS

I'm an ER doc. I care for patients. All patients: Those who need to be in the ER; those who don't; those who wouldn't be there if they knew better. For them, for you and for fun, I've got some tips to keep you happy, safe and away from my ER. Enjoy.

1. **Never, ever say "hold my beer and watch this!"** Besides "I do!" they are the most dangerous words ever spoken. They're a harbinger of disaster worse than "Winter is coming." They have their own section on YouTube – great watch after a rough day. They're better than kittens. Still, hold on to your beer.
2. **NEVER ever drink and drive.** It's obvious, but it's obviously not obvious enough. As per CDC, in 2016, 10,497 people died in alcohol-impaired driving crashes, accounting for 28% of all traffic-

related deaths in the US. They're still counting 2018.

3. **Same with drugs**. Any drugs. Legal, illegal, yours, or borrowed. Except for Tylenol. And Motrin. They're OK.
4. **Don't tell your significant other that your life is no longer worth living,** just to upset them. If they call 911, EMS will bring you to me. I'll keep you until you're legally sober if it takes a week. By the time you're sober, got your evaluation and went home, your significant other has had a chance to enjoy life without you. Speak wisely.
5. **Shoveling the roof is overrated**. Especially in winter. It comes with broken heels, fractured backs, and ER trips. The roof is for the birds. And cats. If you're neither, stay on the ground.
6. **Your motorcycle**? The one you love? I love them too, but I sold mine. My first MCA patient came by ambulance. His leg followed in another car. I'll get a motorcycle when I get terminal cancer. For now, I'll stick with my car. Not your thing? At least wear a helmet.
7. Do not, I repeat, **do not, stick your hand in your snowblower to clean it**. You may never be able to play the guitar or tie your shoes again, and it may put a damper on your loving. Yourself or others
8. **If you've been coughing for a week and you smoke, go buy some honey.** Don't come to the ER unless

you have a fever, you're short of breath or you have chest pain. You'll cough for at least three weeks. There's nothing I can do to stop that unless I kill you. That will stop your cough, but it's illegal.

9. **Your twelve-years-of-God-awful-back-pain? Unless something's really different today, the ER is not the place for it.** Especially now, that Percocet has become a 4-letter word. You'll wait, and wait. You'll get a lot of rotten looks and a script for ibuprofen — 600 mg every 6hrs — or acetaminophen — 650 mg every 6hrs. That's Motrin and Tylenol. Go get them over the counter, and don't overdose.

10. **If you have an appointment with your doctor, don't cancel it to come to the ER** instead because you're too sick to see your doctor. Unless your doctor is Dr. Seuss, Dr. Pepper or a plastic surgeon, caring for sick people is what your doctor does. Keep your appointments.

11. **Don't separate fighting dogs with your bare hands**. Dogs can handle dog bites better than you can. They come from wolves. We come from monkeys. We're out of their league. Stay out of it or use a prop.

12. **Don't throw gasoline on an open flame** unless you're looking for a Brazilian wax.

13. **NEVER EVER stand around minding your own business.** It's one of the most

dangerous things known to man. 90% of my assault victims were doing just that.

14. **Church is dangerous.** That's where my syncopal patients come from. They go to church, they faint, they fall, they break a hip. Bars are safer.
15. **Forget Dr. Google.** He'll drive you insane worrying about improbable things that you can't pronounce, let alone understand, and he won't even give you a work note.
16. If you've already seen a specialist for your problem, **coming to the ER for a second opinion won't help.** I specialize in first opinions.
17. **Unless you're actively trying to reproduce, use condoms.** They are cheaper than medications, alimony, and college. The strawberry ones smell better than diapers.
18. **Get a flu shot.** It beats getting the flu. It won't give you the flu. If you got the flu last time you got a flu shot, it's because they happen in the same season. The flu season.
19. **If you walk with a walker, avoid ladders.**
20. **Turn off your oxygen tank before lighting up.** Even better, stop smoking.
21. **Don't eat spicy food if you have diarrhea.** You'll get sensations like never before. Besides rectal lidocaine – which doesn't feel good – there's little I can do for you. You're going to feel like a reverse fire-spitting dragon. As for

diarrhea: One runny episode doesn't count. Diarrhea is when you run out of toilet paper.
22. **Vaccinate your children**. The connection with autism is fake. The hack who made it up lost his license. Even if it was true – and it's not – I'd rather have an autistic child than a dead one. If you trust Jenny McCarthy more than you trust your pediatrician, you should take your kids to her when they're sick.
23. **Use protection**. Use the guard of your saw. Use safety glasses when you're welding. That's not wimpy – that's smart. Unlike lobsters, you don't regrow limbs, and unlike spiders, you only have two eyes. Use them wisely.
24. **Don't hold your chainsaw between your legs** to start it.
25. **Same with pouring hot coffee.** Set the cup down. It will feel better.

A previous version of this article was initially published 3 March 2019 on RadaJonesMD.com ©RadaJonesMD

THE HEMORRHAGE OF EMERGENCY NURSES

I started my medical career late. Really late. I had already lived a few lives. I had earned a boatload of initials, changed husbands, languages, and continents, I had written a useless novel, and I'd been a Mary Kay lady. One day, as I was looking for something to do with myself, my husband suggested medicine. I spent the next nine years immersed in my medical training, feeling guilty every time I spent time with my family, but I digress.

The day I landed in my new ER, I was on the wrong side of forty. I sported a short copper-red haircut not yet seen in humans and an accent that still takes my patient's mind off their misery (they'll spend their last hard-fought breath to ask where I'm from).

My rural ED is hours north of where people call north. Our winters are long, our people are sturdy, and our geese speak mostly French.

My nurses were guarded at first, but they eventually accepted me in spite of my quirks, hair, accent, and all, and they taught me the ropes:

1. The cold chills are worse than the chills, mainly because the chills don't exist per se. They're either cold or hot, and you'd better figure out which. Cold chills are worser.

2. Eh? is not a question from somebody who can't hear, but a marker of nationality.

3. Bavarian cysts hurt. A lot. They usually grow in the ovaries.

4. When an experienced nurse asks: "Are you sure you want to give that?" you probably don't.

5. If they ask you: "Doctor, would you like to give some vitamin K?" you'd better check the med list for the blood thinners you missed.

6. A "fit" is not trying on a new costume. It's passing out.

7. When a nurse overheads you to a room, get up, and go. Or run away. Whichever's easier.

Twelve years later, my nurses and I had many good shifts and more bad shifts. We saved patients, we lost patients, and we wondered what happened to the patients we lost sight of. We learned to trust each other and have each other's backs, whether we liked each other or not, whether we shared the same patients or not. In my ER, we work in teams - almost like parallel ERs - but when the going gets tough, we all do whatever it takes. I'll go see her patient with a heart rate of 160, even if he isn't mine; she'll come to get an IV in my 2 months old, even if he isn't hers. Like soldiers fighting the same war, we're all on the same side in the fight against death. We muddle our way through shifts, skipping lunch, drinking stale coffee, seeing patient after patient on a full bladder. We get cursed, bit and spat on. We laugh at things ordinary people wouldn't laugh about, just to keep ourselves from crying.

A few years ago, my friends, the ER nurses, started leaving. Some retired. Some moved to winter-friendly places where ice only lives in cocktail glasses. Some went to travel nursing to see the world.

But most of them didn't go far. They went to the ICU, to surgery, to administrative jobs. Few of today's ER nurses were there five years ago. Fewer still were there before me.

The young ED nurses are lovely: dedicated, funny, and smart. They work hard and learn fast. They advocate for their patients, and they're fun to work with. But, unlike my old friends, they haven't been through decades of challenging patients, extreme situations, new doctors. When things don't work as they should, when the patient is like no other, when the doctor's overwhelmed, they're at a loss. How could they not?

How does it feel to be the most experienced person in the room, you ask? Not good.

I miss my old nurses like crazy. When the systolic drops, when you ask for the tracheal hook and are met with blank stares, when nobody knows where the jet ventilator is, wouldn't you like to have somebody who knows better than you?

Why are they leaving? Where are they? I polled them on Facebook. I got a deluge of answers - sad, angry, hopeless - about the state of Emergency Nursing today. Here are a few.

"Lack of resources, lack of support, and reimbursement for continued education, unsafe staff/patient ratios. The ER is the most likely unit to be assaulted.

Patient satisfaction trumps evidence-based practice. I am an educated licensed professional, but I can't have a drink or a cell phone at my workplace. The CEO makes $3.2 million, and I can't afford a 2-bedroom apartment."

"Abuse. At the hands of patients, family, either in the form of physical or psychological harm; RNs are sick of feeling disrespected, unheard and dismissed by doctors; The system is broken. Equipment doesn't work. You have a critical patient who speaks Farsi, and the translation devices don't work, and you can't communicate."

"In the ER, you see the worst side of people and society. You see people in pain and distress, and they lash out at you to "fix" them right now. In our evolving society where instant gratification is becoming more prevalent, people expect to go to the ER and to be given answers for long-term problems. The patients are demanding and want all your attention on them. Our culture caters to those who complain because of fear of a bad review. Management puts more and more demands on nursing staff. We can no longer provide quality, critical thinking care to those in true need for fear of discipline."

"I've been out of nursing for a couple of years. I was watching a show on Asian food. It struck me as odd that it would take this Taiwanese restaurant 6 months training on making the noodles that you find in dim sum. It started me thinking that our local ER gave six weeks training then kicked you out of the nest. Hmmm! I will tell anyone that I would rather stand naked on I-95 than ever return to ER Nursing."

"Patients without true emergencies are seen in climbing numbers and congesting the ER. We are expected to work long hours day after day. Our job is so regimented..... let's not look at the idea that you may have just provided the best hands-on care and saved a

life, but you didn't check this box or this one.... oh and granny down the hall complained you didn't smile. It took FIVE (!!!) Years working there before I was approved a single day off without having to call in sick. You never have a moment to breathe, just keep trucking to the next."

Like it or not, this is Emergency Nursing today. They are overworked, abused, and feel undervalued. They are burned out.

What should we do about this? You, me, the other doctor, the other patient? Whoever you are, this affects you. Your family. Your neighbors. YOU.

What will you do about it?

A version of this article was initially published on 6 Jan 2019 on RadaJonesMD.com @RadaJonesMD

THE ER LAWS

Murphy's Law as it applies to the ER: If something can go bad, it will do so in a hurry. If it can't possibly go bad, it will still find a way.

Clock's First Rule: All the patients will crash at the same time. Usually when the computer system goes down.

Clock's Second Rule: The sickest patients will come just before the shift change.

Haste's Theorem: The healthier the patient is, the more they insist on being seen first. Sick patients are not in a hurry.

Lefty's Corollary: The patient who doesn't ask "When is the doctor coming?" is probably dead.

McDonald's Law: The patient who needs sedation will stop at McDonald's on his way to the hospital.

Sweet's Exception: Unless they are diabetics. Then they didn't eat for three days, but they did get their insulin.

Sandwich's Principle: All vomiting patients request a sandwich.

Mass's Law: Whenever a non-ambulatory patient needs to be moved, he will weigh at least 300 pounds.

Law's First Rule: Every drunk patient has a lawyer on speed dial.

Law's Second Rule: All alcoholics will start withdrawing before becoming legally sober.

Law's Third Rule: Every lawyer in the ED will be *your patient.*

Law's Rule on Charting: The ONE case you documented poorly will turn bad and get you sued.

Urin's First Law: The consultant you paged an hour ago will call back as soon as you go to the bathroom.

Urin's Second Law: All babies will pee as soon as you remove their diaper. On you.

Urin's Third Law: Whenever you need urine, the patient has just peed.

Cutter's Law of Time: The surgeon who performed the surgery is never the one on-call.

Cutter's Law of Space: The surgery was never done at your hospital.

Timer's Law: Whenever you manage to go to see a patient, they just went to radiology.

Gyn's Principle: The pelvic stretcher is always inhabited by a large non-ambulatory male.

The Law of Detrimental Location: The trauma victim was just sitting there minding his own business.

Bleeder's Law of Priority: The most important lab will be the first one to clot and the last to result.

Bleeder's Law of Excruciating Challenge: The

likelihood that the labs will clot again is directly proportional to the difficulty of getting them.

Bleeder's Inevitability Principle: You can't stop the bleeding even if the INR clotted on its way to the lab.

Home's Placement Law: Patients will need placement only after case management has left.

Hitchcock's Theorem: The likelihood of a patient having a long QT is directly proportional to the degree of psychosis.

Middlesex's Law on Gender: If you are female, you are a nurse. If you're male, you are a doctor.

Prick's Principle: The fear of needles is directly proportional to the number of tattoos.

Segway's First Risk Theorem: The likelihood of medical errors increases exponentially in VIPs.

Segway's Second Risk Theorem: The nicer the patient, the worse the disease.

Segway's Corollary: All nice patients will have cancer, a stroke or at least a broken hip.

Segway's Pregnancy Conundrum: Sitting on the toilet or swimming in the pool may get you pregnant.

Initially published 15 Jan 2019 ©RadaJonesMD

DEATH BY PATIENT SATISFACTION

The new Holy Grail of business, Customer Satisfaction — CSAT to her close friends — is a measure of how products and services supplied by a company meet customer expectations. In a marketplace where businesses compete for customers, CSAT is a crucial element of strategy.

Why? Money.

Satisfied customers buy. They come back and buy more. They tell their friends, who'll buy too. If satisfied, they'll return and buy more. That's gold for the bottom line. Hail the almighty dollar!

I'm an ER doc. My customers are my patients. Since American healthcare is a business with its own shaky bottom line, though it looks like a bottomless pit, the rage of customer satisfaction hit us hard.

"Over the past decade the government has fully embraced the "patient is always right" model — these surveys focus on areas like waiting times, pain management and communication skills —

betting that increased customer satisfaction will improve the quality of care and reduce costs. There's some evidence they have. An Obamacare initiative adds extra teeth, to the tune of $850 million, reducing Medicare reimbursement fees for hospitals with less-than-stellar scores…Accordingly, hospitals kowtow to…Press Ganey …helping hospitals fulfill their mandated obligation. Some have taken an extra step, tying physicians' compensation to their ratings," Kai Falkenberg explains in a 2013 Forbes article.

In this profit-driven view, my job as an ER doc is to provide products that my patients can't wait to buy. Some are tangible — Percocet prescriptions, relocated hips, work excuses, removed foreign bodies. Some are intangible, like reassurance: "No, you're not having a heart attack, it's probably heartburn. Your sixth beer didn't sit well on top of those burgers."

My customer-driven focus is to make sure that they're satisfied to come back for more.

"I really hope you enjoy your Percocet. Don't hesitate to return if you need more, I'll be happy to throw in some Dilaudid for your back pain."

"Your rectal foreign body? Please have fun and come back anytime, we're open 24/7."

"Your heartburn? I hope there's some beer left in your fridge! Come back soon!"

"You had a few drinks and hit a tree? No problem! I really enjoyed intubating you. I'd love to do it again soon!

"No, you're not having a heart attack today, but if you keep smoking and stay on a steady diet of donuts and fries, I'll be happy to provide you with the best care for your heart attack! It shouldn't take long!

I'll call that PSER — Patient Satisfaction model of ER care. I'll patent it.

When my customer Mr. P. D. (Percocet Deficient) comes in for his fix, and I provide it, he's satisfied. He'll come back and send his friends. I'll soon have the best satisfaction ratings and the financial benefits that go with them. They'll ask to see me, only me. That's excellent patient satisfaction. Let's do more of it!

Oh, wait! We've already done that! Opioid epidemic, anyone? Remember when the Health Care governing bodies berated doctors for not treating pain? We, doctors, created generations of Americans who'll never walk straight again because of their untreated back pain. JCAHO and CMMS, trained by the Big Pharma, whipped us into prescribing Oxycontin (not addictive). That's over now. Now, we're responsible for the opioid epidemic. But I digress.

There's more to patient satisfaction than opioids.

There's the weak and dizzy. They've been like that for months, years maybe. The family had enough. "You must keep her. She can't live alone. She's been unsteady on her feet for years. If you let her go, her broken hip will be on you. You're also spoiling our dinner plans. You know who I am? You'll find out. What's your name? Jones? Well, Dr. Jones, your CEO is my golf buddy. You won't like what happens to you."

Some need to be seen first. The 21-year-old in alcohol withdrawal. The end-stage fibromyalgia. The 70-year-old in need of Viagra. They need to be seen NOW, or they'll give you a bad review. They're the ones filling in the survey that your pay is based on. They're the ones that matter.

The cardiac arrests? The arrhythmias? The hypotensive sepsis with altered mental status? The anaphylaxis who can't breathe? The STEMI with tombstones on their EKG? They don't count. They don't even know for sure if they're alive or dead, let alone fill in the survey. The dead won't fill them anyhow. Those who survive won't either. ED satisfaction surveys look only at the patients who get directly discharged from the ED - not the sick.

Same with the mental health patients, including the mentally ill children who spend days to weeks in the ED because there isn't a psychiatric bed for them. They linger around like lost souls in Purgatory, bored out of their minds. They occasionally blow up, so we have to restrain and sedate them, but that's OK. They don't fill in the surveys anyhow.

Then there are urgent needs: sandwiches, blankets, sodas, and urinals.

I can't remember a patient asking for epinephrine. Ever. Pepsi? Now you're talking! "Ginger ale? You only have ginger ale? How about Pepsi? No? What sort of ED is this? My wife can't have Ginger Ale, it constipates her! Your sandwiches are stale! Can she have a burger? No? She's hungry! We've been waiting for the CT scan for an hour! She needs to eat!"

Telling him that she'll probably survive another hour without food and that she'd actually benefit from losing a hundred pounds won't help. I've never ever had someone thanking me for telling them to lose weight. No matter how kind I try to be when I tell them that their knees will thank them for losing a few pounds, I can't remember a single one satisfied with my advice.

Same with smoking. "I've heard that a hundred times already, I don't need to hear it again." Yes, you do, if you're still smoking, you do. And telling me that you're on Chantix doesn't make you a non-smoker. It makes you a smoker on Chantix, but that's not important right now. Your satisfaction is.

Does better satisfaction mean a better quality of care? Probably not.

A study published in JAMA in Feb 2013, included data from 52K adults found that the most satisfied patients spent the most on health care (9% more), were more likely to be admitted, and were most likely to die (12.6% more).

Who cares? This isn't about patient safety. It's about patient satisfaction. After all, that's where the money is. Prioritize, will you?

I came up with a plan:

1. We'll start with the patient satisfaction surveys. We'll hand them in in triage with a smile, a handful of Percocets, and a menu.

2. We'll have the triage nurse order their burgers/blankets/Pepsi/nicotine patches as they sign in.

3. We'll wheel them into the room of their choice and we'll make sure to thank them for coming in.

4. Triage should call a Code VIP for every likely-to-survey patient so that we see them first.

As for those who can't fill the surveys, whether it's because they're paralyzed or unconscious or dead — let them wait until they become more reasonable or die. We'll just make sure to provide maximal satisfaction to those who fill in the surveys. That's what it's all about, isn't it? That's where the money is.

Looking forward to the bright future of our American health care. I hope you are too.

Originally published 9 Jan 2019 ©RadaJonesMD

I'M AN ER DOC AND I HAVE NO FRIENDS

Every time I call a friend, all I have for them is more work. I've never yet called to say: "I hope you're having a great day. Why don't you take a break and have some fun? You've worked enough."

Nope. I only call to give them extra work. Whether it's 2AM or 2PM, I need you to get away from your bed/lover/high horse and come take my patient. All, always, sick. The healthy ones I send home without waking you up.

Sometimes they're not sick enough. My ortho friend says: "Are you crazy? Just because she has broken her wrists you think she needs to stay?"

"She walks with a walker. How's she gonna walk? How's she gonna wipe herself? How's she gonna stay alive?"

He looks at me like I've lost it. He doesn't do comfort or supportive care. The patients either need surgery or they don't. It's not rocket science. It's not his problem. But then whose is it?

Sometimes they're too sick. "Are your out of

your mind? She's 95, her systolic is 74 and you want me to admit her to the ICU? Call the hospitalist and make her comfort care."

I'd be happy to, but it's not my call. It's hers. If she's with it and she wants the intubation and the electricity and the broken ribs from CPR, in short, she wants everything done, it's her choice. She'll get everything done, at whatever cost to herself, to her family, to society as a whole. I'm not entitled to make decisions for her even if I think I know better, even if I wouldn't make those same decisions for myself.

It gets even worse when it's the family's decision. Her daughter who left home at 22 and hasn't seen her in 50 years; her ex, who eloped with the babysitter and is now so sorry that he wants EVERYTHING done so he can confess — I mean apologize — and get it off his chest? They want it all, the rib-breaking CPR and the Foley catheter and the tubes, as many of them as her body can stand, and whatever other misery I can inflict on her as long as she gets to stay alive long enough for them to drop their load on her and be set free.

But I digress. I was talking about my friends, the ones I call when the going gets tough and I need help.

I call my cardiologist. "I have this 90-year-old with an EF of 25 who comes complaining of fatigue. Her troponin is 7."

"Why are you calling me?"

"I thought you were the cardiologist."

"So what? There's nothing I can do for her. She gets admitted every week for something. There's nothing I can do for her, why call me?"

I get angry. Very angry.

"She's got a long cardiac history, chest pain, an abnormal EKG and a troponin of 7." I say it softly, as softly as the hissing long fuse of a detonation cord after it's been lit.

"She always makes troponin. She's got to have some arrhythmia; she always makes troponin when she's got an arrhythmia. What's her EKG like?"

"It's sinus at 110. I see no arrhythmia. I can take a picture of it and send it to you."

"No need. I can access her EKG."

Maybe you should, then.

"I'll see her but I won't admit her. Give her to the hospitalist."

Of course. If there's anybody on the totem pole lower than me, getting shat upon every day by every specialty known to man, it's the hospitalist.

They are smart and hardworking and always there. They are the Cinderellas of medicine. Their ugly stepsisters piss on them whenever they get a chance. Not directly, no. Via me. I get to call them and get them to admit surgical patients and oncological patients and cardiology patients and any other patients. Soon enough I'll call them to admit patients for the vet down the road. He's a specialist too. "I have this 2-year old-lizard..."

I call the hospitalist. She has an accent. She came here legally to practice medicine but the system didn't allow her into the hot fields like dermatology, ENT or neurosurgery. She got to be a hospitalist in this after-life, whether she was a Nephrologist in Peru, an Endocrinologist in Romania, or an Oncologist in Bulgaria.

She's smarter than I am— she's an internist. They think long and act slow. I'm an ER doc. I think fast and act now. I'm the cowboy while she's the judge. The house of medicine needs us both.

"Why do you think this patient needs admission?"

"Well, she can't walk," I say, feeling like a fraud.

"Did you try walking her?"

"No. She walks with a walker and now she has two broken wrists."

Or a hip. Or a pelvis. Or something else that's going stop her from going home to her previously marginal function. I can't send her home, and nobody else wants her.

"She's all yours."

Still wondering why I have no friends?

Initially published 19 Jan 2019 ©Rada Jones MD

STRANGEST REAL PATIENT COMPLAINTS, PART 1

---

1. Female patient with lower abdominal pain: "I have a history of Bavarian cysts."

2. Patient with leg swelling coming for an ultrasound: "My doctor said that I may have a blood clog in my leg."

3. Patient with fever and headache: "I have a stiff neck. My doctor said it could be Smiling Mighty Jesus."

4. "My lips are chapped."

5. Triage note: "Patient was attacked by an ostrich."

6. Patient with vaginal discomfort: "I can't get the apple out of my vagina. The orange came out fine last night." The apple had to be surgically removed.

7. "The left side of my brain isn't working, but it gets better when I eat beets."

8. A gentleman with a Superman cape got hit by a car. He came in naked, wearing only his cape and

his socks. His complaint? "The FBI implanted something in my brain, and now I can't fly!"

9. Patient comes in for an animal bite: "I got attacked by a squirrel."

10. Patient with abdominal pain: "I was cleaning my butt with my electric toothbrush, and it got sucked in the whole way."

11. Elderly patient living alone: "Ghosts are sexually assaulting me."

12. Zoo-keeper: "I was cleaning the yak pen, and they attacked me."

13. Patient complaining of a headache: "I was sexually assaulted by the mushrooms I ate. They melted my brain."

14. Agitated female patient: "Ghosts are touching my cat."

15. EMS report: "The patient thinks she's a cat."

16. Triage note: "The patient states he got attacked by vampires."

17. Triage, 3AM on Christmas day: "I'm Jesus Christ. I was told to come to see you."

18. Fifteen years old blonde girl: "I woke up looking like Forest Whitaker."

19. Elderly smoker on oxygen: "My cough got worse. I think I've got ammonia."

20. Young woman opens her mouth wide and points at her throat: "My vulva is swollen."

21. Teenage boy in camouflage pants: "I'm a robot, and my sister put me together wrong. Watch…" He shakes her arms to demonstrate.

22. "My pussy be drippin…"

23. EMS report bringing in a frail elderly patient: "He got blown over by the wind at the waffle house."

Stay Away from MY ER and Other Fun Bits ... 29

24. Tearful teenage girl: "My stuffed animals keep saying, "kill me, bitch."

25. "Every time I ejaculate, I smell like bleach."

26. Patient's boyfriend: "She tastes funny down there."

27. Patient with dysuria: "We had sex, and he went into where I pee. Now it hurts to pee."

28. EMS report: "Two years old fell into Grandfather's grave."

29. Patient coming for a sore throat, pointing to his uvula: "The thing that hangs down in the back of my throat is upside down, and now I can't swallow my spit."

30. Patient brought in by EMS with a tourniquet around his arm: "I cut off my hand, and I threw it in the trash."

31. EMS call: "It's a twofer. The first patients is bleeding from groin trauma. The second patient had a seizure and choked."

32. Post-surgical patient coming for pain: "My surgeon said I could have a hematomato."

33. Patient complaining of pain in his side: "I have a bleeding hemorrhoid." He pulls his shirt to reveal a draining abscess.

34. Triage note: "Glass rod shattered inside the penis."

35. Patient coming for abdominal pain: "I had a vasectomy last week, and now my ovaries hurt."

36. Intoxicated patient brought in by EMS: "I'm feeling homicidal after seeing a midget, a unicorn, a leprechaun, and a dog playing cards..."

37. "I just came to make sure that my dealer gave me the good meth."

38. Call to triage: "Do you pierce baby's ears?"

39. After a sack of flour got spilled outside a

grocery store, the whole town came in to be tested for anthrax.

40. "I'm being controlled like an avatar, and I woke up with a moist butt hole."

41. Patient complaining of testicular discomfort: "I have a worm in my tentacle," he says, pointing to a testicular vein.

42. Triage note: "The patient is here for Gorilla glue in his hair."

43. "I sat on a cocaine-dusted gerbil, and he crawled into my butt. He's trying to claw his way back out, but he got lost, and now I'm bleeding."

44. Triage note: "Patient complaining of a sore throat after drinking cleaner fluid."

45. "I got food stuck in my sarcophagus."

46. "Google said I could die from hypothermia, so I wanna make sure I'm not too cold." 98F.

47. "I burned my finger on a French Fry, and I need Dilaudid."

48. "I have acid reflex."

49. EMS report: "The patient called an ambulance because she dreamed she had a stroke."

Initially published 4 Feb 2019 ©RadaJonesMD

PUT ME TO SLEEP

The heavy young man curled on his left side is in the ER for a pain in his backside. The sweaty blue dragon on his chest smells like fear.

"It's an abscess. I'll have to open it. It will hurt."

"Can you put me to sleep? I hate pain."

I can. Should I? Remember Michael Jackson? I do.

My patient's neck would make a Hereford bull proud; he's missing a chin but he's got a 7-month sized pregnant belly. Intubating him would be a challenge on a good day, and this isn't one of those since he needs to lay face-down for the procedure.

"Sorry, no can do. Putting you to sleep is a bad idea. You may never wake up again."

The 40-year-old grandma with purple lipstick and a week of left-hand numbness has a hint of beer on her breath. She says her doctor sent her to get an MRI. She wants it now, otherwise my Press Gaineys will plummet. So will my paycheck. I'll have to live on Cheerios for a month, and they aren't low carb.

"I can't get into that machine. You'll have to put me to sleep."

I don't think so, my friend. The MRI is a bad place to have a code. If you stop breathing while you're in there, your numbness may be gone forever but so will the rest of you. They won't even notice that you're dead. Put you to sleep? Not me, not today.

Then there's this cute chubby toddler. She hasn't used her left hand since she tripped and her mom held her up. She's playing on Mom's phone, happy as can be.

"Her elbow's out. It's called a nursemaid's elbow. I'll have to twist her arm to get it back. She's going to scream like a banshee, but it will be over in seconds."

Mom chokes. "Can you put her to sleep?"

I feel for you, I really do, but the answer is no. It's too risky to put her to sleep for a 5-second procedure she'll never remember in order to save you this pain. So sorry. No.

The old folks are the hardest to say no to. They want no part of the life that's left to them, whether it's in their own lonely home or at the nursing home where the kids dropped them off. They're not demented — I can't remember a single demented patient asking me to kill them. They're just too weak to kill themselves.

"Can you put me to sleep so that I never wake up? Please? I'm 87, I've got nothing left to live for. My wife died last year and the kids are gone. I'm all alone. I can't even pee by myself. I hate my life, I hate the nursing home, you can't send me back there, please, you wouldn't do that to a dog!

You're right sir, I wouldn't do that to a dog, but you're not a dog. You are a human being and therefore entitled to an unspecified amount of suffering, an endless amount of loneliness, and the privilege of rotting in your own urine for as long as it will take you to die in a medically acceptable manner. I can't take that away from you. Not only would I lose my license, which is important to me, but I'd end up in jail — remember Dr. Kevorkian?

As for the dog, you are correct. It so happens that I have an old dog. Her flowing lupine leaps that I so loved are a thing of the past. She now falls over whenever her back legs fail. Cataracts cloud her loving eyes and she struggles to find her frisbee. She often needs my touch to remember who and where she is. I watch her. I listen to her. "Are you loving your food?" I cook for three since dog food is for dogs, not for her. Tonight it's chicken breast with corn and peaches. "Are you still enjoying your short walk and your even shorter swim? Do you still greet me every morning like I'm the sun, telling me that it's going to be a wonderful day since we're together? Are you still enjoying life?"

When the answer will be no — any day now — I'll do for her what I wish somebody will do for me. I'll hold her lovingly and help her through the rainbow bridge as I'm dying inside.

As for you, my old, lonely, hopeless friend, I can't help you. Unless I'm ready to give up my profession and my freedom, I can't help you. In America, mercy killing is killing.

Please, please get your advanced directives and talk to your proxy, will you? And never sign up for a DNI without a DNR.

Hang in, my friend. The end is near.

Initially published Aug 2018 ©RadaJonesMD

13 REASONS TO CHOOSE A WOMAN DOCTOR

Like all doctors, I'm a lousy patient. My doctor is a lovely man, but going to see him? That's right there with weighing myself, getting a flu shot and doing my taxes, and behind celebrating Thanksgiving with the in-laws and getting a root canal.

And I'm not the only one. If I had a dollar for every patient who told me they hate doctors (no offense), I'd be long retired.

If you're like us, I have a tip for you. Choose a woman doctor.

Why?

1. **You'll be more likely to survive a heart attack.** Female doctors have lower patient mortality and readmission rates. To me, that matters, since I hate hospital food and I detest going to funerals.
2. **They don't wear ties**. Ties are relics. They belong with the dinosaurs. They indicate that the wearer is somebody. In

doctors, that's somebody covered with germs. A tie is Noah's ark for germs looking for a home. Don't let that home be you.

3. **They listen longer.** Today's doctors are too busy to listen to their patients. The average male doctor interrupts a patient after 47 seconds, but female doctors will let you speak for three whole minutes.

4. **They tend to be more thorough**. Whenever my husband cleans the kitchen, there's stuff left for me to do. He's good with the big picture – but the details? He doesn't see the breadcrumbs. I do. Women doctors are more likely to deal with every detail and leave no loose ends.

5. **Men compartmentalize better, women are better at multitasking**. Your woman doctor will remember your blood pressure, your work note, and the script for Viagra even if her pager goes off, the Patriots won, and she's late for dinner.

6. **They are more likely to follow guidelines.** That's good, since guidelines are evidence-based and meant to improve your medical care.

7. **They communicate better, providing patient-centered care.** Instead of just telling you what to do, they'll work with you to get you the care you need.

8. **They're more likely to include your family in your care.**

9. **They have smaller hands.** Why does that matter? Try getting a pelvic or a

rectal exam from somebody built like a linebacker, and you'll understand.
10. **They'll counsel you on your health behaviors**. They'll work with you on stopping smoking, losing weight or drinking less. You don't want to hear that. Neither do I. But a healthy lifestyle will help you live longer and improve your quality of life.
11. **They provide better quality of care in diabetes.**
12. **They provide emotional support.** So do men doctors, of course. Still, it's not the same. I hug my patients when I feel they need it. My male colleagues give fist bumps. And so they should, these days when everything can be construed as sexual. Fist bumps work for toddlers, but not when giving someone bad news.
13. **Women always wash their hands after they pee.**

Initially published 21 Oct 2019 ©RadaJonesMD

VOMIT: VICTIMS OF MODERN INFORMATION TECHNOLOGY

Doctors take notes. So do nurses. They don't have a choice. Documentation comes with the job, and it takes more time than actually seeing patients. Whether you like it or not - I hate it - it's part of the job. Insurance companies and trial lawyers say that whatever didn't get documented didn't happen.

That's bullshit. I do things that I never document all the time. Like food. I didn't document my food intake – no matter what the scale says – but it somehow happened, given the 10 extra pounds on my cruise East. I never documented having sex, but I have a 31-years old who says he's my son. He's got my crooked fingers to prove it.

So, things happen, if you document them or not. However, that doesn't count in a trial. If you're in healthcare, documenting is part of your job, whoever you are. It often hurts, and it always impacts patient care. It didn't use to be so.

First came the SOAP notes. They had nothing

to do with cleanliness. Just the opposite. SOAP stood for: Subjective, Objective, Assessment and Plan.

S: "Patient states that pain is 16/10, sharp, unremitting. Feeling like a crocodile is eating his insides every 10 minutes, after sprinkling them with Frank's hot sauce."

O: On entering the room, patient is eating Cheetos and drinking Mountain Dew while texting. Abdomen is soft and non-tender.

A: Abdominal pain, probably gastritis.

P: Remove Cheetos, offer Maalox, follow up with PCP.

Next came the T sheets. Things changed. Instead of me deciding what to write, the form prompted me through questions, some relevant, some not.

"Tell me about your shortness of breath," I'd ask.

"I'm not short of breath. I'm here for a penile discharge, but I didn't want to tell them in triage."

Unrelenting progress and Obamacare brought us the blessing of EHR, Electronic Health Records. Now, my computer harasses me into documenting everything, relevant or not. That allows the hospital to charge for it. Money? That's always relevant.

The EHR system rules my life, eats my lunch and inhabits my nightmares. It's a match made in hell. Like a nagging partner, it incessantly spits nasty little comments to stop me in my tracks.

"Temperature."

"103."

EHR turns pink, ignoring my efforts to save my documentation. I may notice it. I may not.

If I don't, I'm screwed. I get to start over.

Stay Away from MY ER and Other Fun Bits ...

If I do, I go back and I find the pink box.

1. C/F.

C is Celsius. I know Celsius. I love Celsius. I was born in Celsius. It's a wonderful system with crystal clear limits. Water freezes at zero. Water boils at 100. That's it.

Easy, no?

I don't know about other doctors, but I have a short supply of boiled patients. Mine usually come raw. At 103, they'd be seriously overcooked.

I know that. My nurses know that. Even my stethoscope knows that.

My computer doesn't. It forces me back through documenting senseless boxes.

My patients wait. My patients leave. My patients die.

Without me. I'm busy, spending quality time with EHR.

103.

C/F.

F.

Moving on. Next: Pain.

Continuous? Intermittent? Fluctuant? Radiating? Waxing? Waning? Occasional? Sharp? Dull? Achy? Burning? Crampy?

Like, really?

If they can speak, and *if* they have their hearing aids on, and *if* they are neither drunk, nor obtunded, or on the phone with somebody more important than me, our conversation goes something like this:

"When you got dizzy, how did that feel?"

Suspicion ensues. For full disclosure: I have an

accent. I sound like Dracula. My friends call it my Beekmantown accent.

"Like, dizzy. "

"Say I never heard the word 'dizzy' before. How would you explain it to me?"

They look at their spouse. They consider bolting. They give me another chance.

"I was like, dizzy."

"Dizzy like passing out, or dizzy like the room is spinning?"

"Dizzy like dizzy. "

Take that, EHR. Pain, like, pain. It hurts.

We're moving on to the physical exam. We document.

"The abdomen is: Soft? Hard? Tympanitic? Obese? Scaphoid? Distended?

The discharge is: Clear? Serosanguinolent? Bloody? Purulent? Scant? Abundant?

I spend more than three-quarters of my shift on the computer, trying to document. Another 10% communicating with my staff. Another 10% on the phone, advertising my patients to consultants as if I'm trying to sell them a used car.

Everything else is direct patient care. How's your math?

To be fair, I do type like a Neanderthal — I hope that's not a racist comment - yet. My younger colleagues have nimble fingers, dancing on the keyboard like ballerinas performing Swan Lake. Mine? Two old drunks trying to waltz.

Done documenting? Time to put in orders. EHR is there, standing right between my patients and my care.

"Aspirin, 325," I try to order.

Stay Away from MY ER and Other Fun Bits ... 43

EHR turns deep pink and balks. "Allergy to Aspirin."

I click on it, trying to find out what that is.

"Stomach upset."

I click the next button, looking for: "That's not a fucking allergy." It's not there.

I shrug and click "medically necessary".

I go to the next order: "Ciprofloxacin."

My EHR gets really upset. "Not indicated in pregnancy."

Pregnancy?! She's 55! Really?

I log out and I go back to my patient.

"Any chance you may be pregnant?"

She looks at me like I've lost it.

"I'm 55. I had a hysterectomy 12 years ago."

I smile and nod, then go back to EHR. I scan in my ID, then type in my username, my password, my PIN.

That's no good.

I start over.

I get it right this time. I log in. I look for: "not pregnant."

It's not there. I shrug and click:

"Medically indicated."

It's the same with lactation.

EHR must think that humans, since they are mammals (unlike factory-built computers,) once pregnant, stay pregnant. Indefinitely. Unless they start lactating. Then they lactate forever, like goats. I disagree.

EHR doesn't care.

"Medically indicated."

Done with the orders.

I finally get to medical decision making, the

most important part of the chart. The part that really matters. That, I can input as I choose.

I skip it.

I've been fighting EHR for an hour now for this one patient while many others are waiting. I hope they didn't die yet.

Here's to VOMIT — Victims of Modern Information Technology in the ER.

Initially published 6 Jan 2019 ©RadaJonesMD

RECYCLE THYSELF

BBC: "*Jemima Layzell, a 13-year-old girl who died from a brain aneurysm has helped...eight different people, including five children, through organ donation...no other donor had helped as many people. Jemima collapsed during preparations for her mum's 38th birthday party and died four days later... Her heart, small bowel, and pancreas were transplanted into three different people while two people received her kidneys. Her liver was split and transplanted into a further two people, and both of her lungs were transplanted into one patient. Normally, a donation results in 2.6 transplants.*"

As I got older, I stopped worrying about looking good – it never worked anyhow, and now it's too late. I started thinking more about my spare parts. They aren't pretty, and they don't smell good, (I learned that in Surgery,) but they keep me alive. My kidneys relieve me of my half-gallon of morning coffee, my liver lets me enjoy a glass of wine (or two), and thanks to my corneas and my many reading glasses, I can read, write, watch TV.

Like the matching gears of a well-oiled machine, your organs are essential to your life. Except for two: Your gallbladder – her life-goal is to make you crave French Fries and donuts, then shrink your clothes when you aren't watching. And your appendix. He was invented to wake up grumpy surgeons and get you irradiated with CTs. But I digress.

Your organs let you enjoy life. Thanks to their good behavior, you can breathe well enough to make it to your grandkids' soccer game, you can have a beer without drowning your lungs and you can enjoy a burger without turning yellow.

Some are not so lucky.

My patient L., a woman in her thirties, died slowly. She came back week after week, so I can drain the fluid from her abdomen to help her breathe, after alcohol had killed her liver.

After his heart attack, G.'s heart started failing. He was 58. His heart didn't have the strength to pump the blood out of his soggy lungs. They filled with fluid. His breathing suffered. He barely walked to the bathroom. He couldn't lay flat, so he slept in a recliner on the good days when he was home. Those days got fewer and fewer.

M, a beautiful woman in her twenties, was pregnant. Her kidneys had been iffy for a while. Her pregnancy didn't help. A second pregnancy put her on the transplant list. There were no matches but her mother. She got rejected because her tests weren't good enough. M. waited and waited on the transplant list, wondering what would happen to her kids.

Let's talk transplant. That's getting refurbished with other people's spare parts. Like fixing a car, except we're talking new lungs instead of new breaks. Taking parts from the dead to fix the live ones? No brainer! Well, it's a brainer. Transplants are difficult. Transplants are expensive. Transplants are restrictive.

Organs are scarce. As per UNOS, on March 9th 2019, there were 113710 people waiting for an organ. Mostly kidneys, followed by livers and hearts. The waiting times vary widely. The average wait for an eight-year-old needing a kidney was 920 days. Every day, twenty people die waiting. Every 10 minutes, another person is added to the waiting list. Still, people take their organs with them, when they die.

Does God need your organs? Apparently not. As per organdonor.gov, most religions allow organ donation *"Organ, eye, and tissue donation is considered an act of charity and love, and transplants are morally and ethically acceptable to the Vatican. (Pope John Paul II, Evangelium Vitae, no. 86)"*.

In the US, you need the donor's consent to use their organs, no matter how dead they are. Even though God may need their soul, but probably doesn't need their heart.

In Europe, twenty-four countries operate under presumed consent. Unless you opt out, your organs are available for somebody who needs them more. Spain is #1, with 35.1 donors per million population, compared to 26 per million in the US.

In China, the organs of executed prisoners are available for transplant. Since their consent is questionable, this practice is widely condemned. I'm a pragmatist. A dead person does not need a liver. Consent? Have they consented to be executed? If you don't need consent to kill people, do you need consent to take their liver? Is the societal good enough to compensate for the harm of the individual? Is there harm done by removing a dead person's liver? What if that person's liver results in cash for the Chinese government? Some say that death row prisoners get executed on command, to provide an organ for an approved match. This is a can of worms I'm not competent to handle. Others have. Ethicists, philosophers, politicians.

Selling human organs is illegal in most of the world. Not so in Iran and the Philippines. Forbes: <u>Selling Your Organs: Should it be Legal? Do You Own Yourself?</u> "there is evidence that the financial incentive works. Organ sales are permitted in the Philippines as long as the donor recipients are natives. A Filipina organ recipient says: "Nobody would donate a kidney without getting paid." Iran uses a hybrid system… vendors sell their organs to the government, which acts as an intermediary. It pays them and gives them free health insurance for one year. Donor recipients must be Iranian and they are required to work to pay for the cost of their organs. The system has virtually wiped out the waiting lists."

This opens the door to organ trafficking. People whose kids are starving may sell parts of themselves in order to feed them, supplying the black market.

How does one find human organs though? How much do they cost? I googled "Human organs for sale." eBay responded: "Organs For Sale Sold Direct – eBay – Fantastic Prices on Organs for Sale." I clicked. "Nord C2 Organ Keyboard synthesizer in excellent condition." No good. I tried again. I came up with: "Kidney for Sale by Owner: Human Organs, Transplant. Preowned." $4.48. Cheap, I thought, but it was just a paperback.

According to Havocscope.com, Global Black-Market information, the asking price for a lung in Europe is $312.650 (you'd think they'd quote it in Euros and round a bit.) The average price paid for a kidney is $150K. Out of that, $5K goes to the kidney provider. The rest is shared between the middlemen.

Aljazeera: *"The illicit kidney trade... has exploded as brokers use social media to find donors. This gaping hole between demand and the legal supply of kidneys is being filled by ...the world's biggest black market for organs, which crisscrosses India, Nepal, Bangladesh, Pakistan, Sri Lanka, and Iran."*

The black market is, by definition, unregulated. Many donors found themselves penniless, without a kidney and without recourse. As always, the poor, the uninformed, the vulnerable.

In our society, you can't pay for organs. You can pay for insurance, for hospitalization, for cancer treatment. You pay for food. Not for organ donation. That's done for love. How many people do you love enough to give them a kidney? The lack of a legal market leads to functional organs being discarded, to sick people dying while waiting for them, and to a thriving black market praying on the vulnerable.

Legalizing organ markets would actually save money in healthcare. ABS-CBN news: *"Kidney transplant patients... enjoy a better quality of life... It is also cheaper...The cost of kidney dialysis in the US averages about $44,000 per year per patient...Separate studies conducted by the UMMC and the Washington University School of Medicine in St. Louis indicate that* *the "break-even" cost of kidney transplants is shrinking. The Washington University School of Medicine study stated that, given reduced transplantation and post-transplantation costs, society could pay each donor $90,000 and easily break even."*

No can do. Selling organs is not ethical. Is selling antibiotics, vaccines, epinephrine, ethical? It's legal! How is selling organs different? It's legal to bury – or cremate – your heart, liver, corneas, after you crushed your brain in a motorcycle accident or overdosed on Fentanyl. Is it ethical? What if there's a mother watching her kid die, in need of a heart? How about the husband hoping a kidney for the mother of his two kids? How about the parents waiting for a match for their toddler? What if this was your kid?…your mom?… your wife?

How about recycling myself, I thought. I looked it up. My chances are mixed – kidneys and lungs look good, but my heart's too old. Thankfully, she doesn't know it. If I want to recycle, I'd better die soon, and die healthy.

In a world where we recycle beer bottles, we make old clothes into quilts and remake the same movies, how about ultimate recycling? How about recycling yourself? I don't know about you, but I love looking at houses for sale. I'm obsessed with traveling. I dream of alternative lives. Who would I be if I was born in Peru, petting llamas? In Portugal, fishing for octopus in clay pots? In Egypt, drinking mint tea instead of wine?

What if my heart got to live again, beating inside the bony chest of a teenager for his first kiss? Inside a mother holding her child? Inside a bride? Would it add to the joy of the universe? Would my spirit soar? Maybe not.

But even if I won't be there to enjoy it, the recipient would. So would her family, her friends, her dog. So would my husband and my son. They'd know that somewhere in the world, my heart still beats, and loves them still. They may feel less alone.

Are you in? If so, what should you do?

1. Tell your family. They need to hear it from you, not from some stranger asking them for your heart before it even got to stop.
2. Start here. They'll redirect you to your state site. Like fish, guests and French baguettes, organs go stale in a hurry. The closer the recipient, the better the results.
3. Live well. Be happy. Be generous and kind. Live as if death can't touch you.

But if the day comes…If that car comes too fast…if that floor is too slippery…if tomorrow never comes…Won't it be good to have your heart love again in somebody's chest? See the world through somebody's eyes? Piss somebody else's beer?

Initially published 10 March 2019 ©RadaJonesMD

WHY I NEVER TELL PEOPLE I'M A DOCTOR

I'm an ER doc and proud of it. But I never mention it when I meet new people. Unless someone's fixing to die, I avoid it like the plague. "I work in a hospital," I say. "Where in the hospital?" "The ER. How about you?" That's always a topic changer since most people would rather talk about themselves.

Why not own it, you ask? There's no shame in being a doctor. It's not like you're a lawyer. I'm not a bank robber, a spammer, or a pimp. Not even a politician. So why avoid it?

First, I hate showing off. As a communist kid, I learned that bragging is a sin, worse than stealing. Whatever belonged to the State belonged to us, the people. So we took it home. They said that a neighbor working at the bike factory stole spare parts to build a bike. Everybody laughed when he ended up with a gun. Not because he was a thief. Because he didn't know what he stole. Unlike my cousin, Decebal, who got a cop drunk, then stole his K9 and sold it to the highest bidder.

Still, bragging was a no-no, and telling people I'm a doctor feels like bragging. After all, how can they up me one? Be a rocket surgeon? The POTUS? Kim Kardashian?

But more importantly, **telling people I'm a doctor never leads to any good.**

Being a doctor makes me an outsider when I'm trying to blend. Like everyone else, I'm more than my job. I'm a mother, a so-so cook, and a pathetic singer. I'm just one of the girls. But, as soon as I admit that I'm a doctor, I'm no longer one of them. Unless I happen to be at a doctor's conference.

After fifteen years of ER, it got old to have people teach me about it. Beauticians, bakers, dog walkers – they can't resist telling me about the show. Sex in the closets? Pen tracheostomy? Shocking asystole? They got it down pat. Even my mother-in-law.

No matter what I do, I'll never be as smart as Dr. Google, who can diagnose everyone. It's bad enough to have my own patients google their symptoms, then teach me about their unique disease, but getting that at a party? Thanks to Dr. Google and TV drug ads, many healthy people find themselves a disease even if doctors can't.

People want free advice, but my insurance says no. Over drinks, during a show, or when trying on shoes, my new friends share their symptoms, and their hairdresser's diagnosis. Then they ask me what I think. What I think? Try Dr. Google.

People want prescriptions. If I'm lucky, it's for

antibiotics. They need a Z-pak, since nothing else works for their cough. When I'm less fortunate, they want Percocet, Xanax or Ambien. The good stuff that will warm up a social gathering.

In my spare time, I get to see things I'd rather not. You like rashes? Neither do I. Not mine, not others'. And they are never on the face, or on the hands. They're always on some secret body part that should stay hidden to all but loving eyes, not uncovered to me in the elevator.

As soon as they hear I'm a doctor, people treat me like I'm rich, expecting me to foot the bill. From tag sales to used cars, I get special doctor prices.

I'm a godsend for the doctor haters, and there are many. Whether their loved one died, they didn't get into medical school, or the damn urologist expects them to pay their bill, it's my fault. The chronic back pains and fibromyalgias – they live to meet me.

I invariably get unpaid work on vacation. Medical emergencies on the plane – no fun after two glasses of wine, especially with antediluvian, German-only medical kits. Hemorrhoids in Peru? Diarrhea in Easter Island? Erectile dysfunction in Thailand? All mine.

When everything is said and done, **being a doctor isn't that much of a crown.** Not even at home. My 30 year old son called to tell me he had chest pain. Should I go to the ER? No, I said. He did anyhow. Was I upset? No. Was I relieved? Yes. Did I feel vindicated when he said: You were right? You betcha!

Initially published 28 Aug 2019 ©RadaJonesMD

HEALTHCARE COSTS AND THE PROVIDER CURSE

My friend, the hospitalist, was livid as he came from meeting the administration. That's not new, he seldom looks happy to see me, but this time he wasn't angry with me.

"They said doctors cost too much!" he sputtered. "We're an expense. An expense the hospital can no longer support. WE are an expense!"

He turned purple. Beautiful color, if you happen to be a Bordeaux. I worried about his blood pressure. He can't have a healthy lifestyle - none of us does. Seven twelves in a string will do a number on your workout routine, your family life, and your sanity.

"I wanted to ask: Why do you think patients come here? To see you? To see what you concoct while sitting in your office popping M&Ms? No! They are here to see doctors. We, doctors, care for the patients. We make you money. It's OUR work that gets YOU paid! And we cost too much?"

To that I'll add: When was the last time YOU saved a life? It still matters a little.

Medicine changed. Remember the family doctor driving his horse-drawn buggy for home visits? Delivering children, letting blood, and getting paid in chickens and honey? Neither do I.

That was BOE. Before our era. Before hospitals, insurance companies, EHR, and Obamacare. Those doctors are dead, lucky them.

You and I, we live in the Provider Era. We are no longer doctors. In our sick healthcare system, we became providers.

"Code 99. Provider Jones to Room 3. STAT."

Cows provide milk. Pigs provide bacon. Farmers provide corn. What do I provide? Percocet? I&Ds? Work notes? How about you? And BTW, which provider school did you go to?

Downgrading doctors to providers was a smart move. It trimmed our aura, downsized our hubris, and reduced our influence. Our expectations and our pay too. It helped bend us to the regulations our administrators exist to enforce. Unless it's the other way round, and regulations only exist for administrators to have something to implement. After all, they need to do something, and they aren't into touching patients.

We're blessed with administrators for every taste. CEOs. COOs. Quality coordinators. Facility planners. Compliance officers. Human resource managers. Risk managers. Trauma coordinators. Patient care advocates. Coders. Education specialists. I'll keep it short here, since some of us actually have to work.

They wear suits. We wear scrubs. They smell like aftershave and cologne. I smell like patients

and stress sweat. They talk Medicalese. I talk ER. Their job is to tell us what to do. Like:
- Fill out ALL forms.
- Check ALL the boxes on ALL the charts.
- Obey the latest genius rule hatched by CMMS.
- Give antibiotics even before we know if somebody's sick.
- Kiss JCAHO's cheeks.
- Have no drinks at the desk. Coffee, I mean. What were you thinking?
- Give drugs to those who say they have pain.
- NO! STOP! Don't give them drugs! You'll make them all into addicts!
- Be nice to patients. They're always right, even when they bite.
- Any spiritual beliefs we need to be aware of? Do they need a shaman? Get a shaman.
- Do they need a translator? They speak English? So what? Ask anyhow.

Thanks to the administrators' care, no patient with a stubbed toe fails to get his religious beliefs recorded, his drinking habits evaluated, and his spiritual needs cared for.

We are the Touchables. Nurses, Doctors, PAs, NPs, CAs. We touch patients: their bodies, their lives, their deaths. We are the ones who tell them that their mother died, their kid has drowned, their husband will never walk again. We tell them that they're dying. We put a stethoscope on their chest, a hand on their shoulder, a finger in their rectum, a tube down their throat. We hug them if they let us.

They touch us. They touch our souls - we spend sleepless nights wondering if another doctor could have saved them. They touch our bodies -they hug us; they punch us; they cut us with the blade they hid in their bra. Our scrubs and our minds are forever stained with their urine, their blood, their sorrow. We inhale their smell, their viruses, their misery.

We're expendable. We're on the frontline in the war against death.

Administrators are a different breed. They don't touch patients. They don't draw blood, they don't clean poop, they don't get hurt. They don't lose their jobs when things go wrong. They have scapegoats. Us.

Over the last two decades, administrators proliferated like mushrooms after a good rain. So did our healthcare spending. Any correlation, you think?

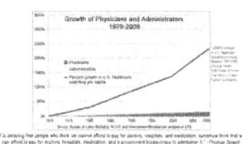

You can't swing a dead cat without hitting a hospital administrator these days. That's comforting as long as you have enough dead cats.

As for doctors? Unless you're bleeding to death, you'll have to wait for months and moths for an endoscopy. I had to pull strings to get one for my husband. It took a month. The same long waits for neurology, urology, ENT, ortho, and any other specialty that I can think of.

Sadly, we have moved very far away from the time when those who touch patients made decisions for their care. Whole armies of administrators exist only to interfere with our care. To deny patients the studies, the admissions, the procedures, and the medications that they need, in order to save money for insurance companies.

We're trapped in a net of rules and regulations compiled and enforced by a growing number of well-paid administrators who will do anything to keep their job. Anything but touch a patient.

Something's rotten in America's healthcare.

Initially published 27 Sept 2019 ©RadaJonesMD

STRANGEST REAL PATIENT COMPLAINTS, PART 2

---

1. Overweight female patient: "I'm tired of my thighs touching."

2. "I'm allergic to tazers."

3. Triage note: "Testicular bleeding. Patient states he stapled his scrotum back together after his spouse lacerated it."

4. Patient BIBA (brought in by ambulance): "I'm bleeding from a paper cut."

5. Elderly gentleman with urinary retention: "I always have problems with my prostitute."

6. Young mother holding her infant: "My son's penis is too small."

7. Patient comes in for fever while bird flu is in the news: "I went to KFC, and I think I caught the bird flu."

8. Triage note: "The patient was brought from jail for drinking from his colostomy bag."

9. Elderly lady coming for a vaginal discharge: "I have purple stuff coming out my lady pocket."

Her husband admits that they ran out of KY jelly and used Smucker's grape jelly instead.

10. Patient with breast pain: "I ripped my nipple with my piercing in the shower."

11. Triage note: "The patient got hit in the face with a catfish."

12. Young man BIBA: "I have a low sperm count."

13. Intoxicated patient brought in from the local bar: "I think someone peed in my beer."

14. "My poop doesn't float."

15. Female patient with vaginal discharge: "My BF said I taste funny." She had trichomonas.

16. Elderly woman getting ready for a rectal: "My husband's usually the one doing this!" "Grandma!" Patient: "I mean getting sick and coming to the ER."

17. Patient coming for vaginal bleeding: "I've got clogs coming out my Eucharist!"

18. Triage note: "Vacuum cleaner stuck on penis."

19. "I accidentally swallowed half a bottle of Clorox bleach."

20. "My penis shrinks when I sneeze."

21. Call to triage: "My child swallowed bathwater."

22. Elderly patient asking for Viagra: "I don't last as long in bed as I used to."

23. "I have a condom lost in my vagina."

24. Patient with left-sided abdominal pain: "I have lickulitis. I need that pill flagall."

25. Hypertensive patient sent in by his PCP: "My doctor said that my diabolic blood pressure is too high." His diastolic was 150.

26. Hypoglycemic patient: "I have diabetes type

Stay Away from MY ER and Other Fun Bits ... 65

3. The one that you fix by eating a candy bar. Type two is the one with a pump. Type one is the one that gets the shots."

27. Triage note: "Patient states that he just doesn't feel like himself."

28. "I got beat up by a ghost."

29. Triage note: "A raccoon fell into the baby stroller at midnight while they were fishing."

30. Female patient with abdominal pain: "I googled it and I'm afraid it's prostate cancer!"

31. Patient: "My pussy hurts." Triage nurse: "We don't treat animals here."

32. "Doc, I have Driver Triculitis."

33. EMS report: "Patient states she has end-stage fibromyalgia."

34. "I brushed my teeth with my hair remover."

35. Triage note: "Patient states he got attacked by an owl."

36. "I can't pee since the aliens froze my urethra."

37. "I didn't smoke anything. But I walked through meth, and it got absorbed through a wound I had on my foot."

38. Patient with cough and fever: "I think I have Flumonia." She had both.

39. "I can't read."

40. Elderly patient looking tired: "I have no ambition." The troponin came back positive. He had a heart attack.

41. Patient with food poisoning: "I'm vomicking out of both ends."

42. Patient with generalized pain: "I have sick as hell anemia."

43. Post-op patient coming in for bleeding:

"The doctor took my castrator out." He was post-prostatectomy.

44. Triage note: "The patient states he has a glass Christmas ornament in his butt." In July.

45. Patient with vaginal bleeding: "I have fireballs in my Eucharist!" I thought she was psychotic, until my nurse explained that she had uterine fibroids.

46. "I was impregnated by my ex-husband, who is a warlock through the internet."

47. Patient with headache and blurry vision: "I got hit in the head by a cow." She was diagnosed with retinal detachment.

48. "My house smells like carbon monoxide."

49. "I knocked my joint out and now can't find it."

Initially published 4 Feb 2019 ©RadaJonesMD

SEX AND THE SILVER FOXES

If you're sexy, fit, and agile, if you can part your thighs and bend your knees, if you can see your private parts without a mirror, ignore this. Move on. This is not for you.

This is for those with flailing sex-drive and failing abilities whose sex life is a challenge, but they'd like to make their partners happy and have some fun. Maybe your parents or grandparents. This must be an awful thought, but I'm pretty sure they did it before, or you wouldn't be here.

Sex in the elderly is not a need. It's a privilege.

Most days, you just hope for a good bowel movement. You walked out of bed, you peed without a tube in your urethra, you pooped without an enema! Wow!

Towards the end of your life, the day you even think about sex is a good day. You have a spring in your step and tickle in your nether parts, reminding you of the good old days. You feel naughty. But your partner…They may or may not be into it.

You're not quite sure how to ask. There used to be signals: that unique smile; that slow touch; the tongue maybe? You didn't use to have dentures, then.

It's hard, whether you've been together forever or just since your granddaughter hooked you up on Tinder. You spoon while you sleep. You switch plates at dinner. Sometimes you take his meds. Your intimacy is not sexual.

Today, you feel the stir. You're not sure how to go there. Wouldn't that be fun?

Maybe.

There are challenges. Artificial hips and fused backs hinder your mobility and limit position choices. Avoid low chairs. They make hips come out, and nothing spoils the mood like an ambulance trip.

Atrophic vaginas lack flexibility, so lubrication is essential. Lubricants come flavored in endless choices. Naked strawberry. Pina Colada. Cinnamon roll. I'm looking for one in bacon. They say bacon makes everything better. You need lube, love, and lots of patience.

The penis needs blood to engorge. Lots of it. Your heart needs to stand up to the challenge, besides just keeping you alive. Sex may be the only demanding physical activity you've engaged on since fighting for that TV on Black Friday. Sex is risky for your heart, your brain, your aorta. Your body works as hard as if you shoveled snow, but you're having too much fun to notice the warnings.

I'm an ER doc, so I've seen plenty of heart attacks and strokes caused by sex. A few deaths. All men. Their lovers were distraught. So were their wives, when they all met at the bedside. I saw that twice. Neither man made it.

Be careful. Speak to your doctor. Ask them if your heart is healthy enough for sex.

Viagra works. It made a difference in my patients' sex lives. It gave them hope and joy. It also gave them HIV, and Hep C. Viagra doesn't work well with alcohol. You may want to forgo the wine and stick with roses and candles. Viagra interferes with nitroglycerin, our go-to drug for the heart, so if you end up in the ER, tell your doctor about it.

Regardless, sex is fun, sex is joy, sex is love. If you're not doing it, you're missing out.

If you're lucky, you have an interested partner. Still, coordinating is a challenge. Maybe it's not their day.

In comes oral sex. The blow job is the refuge of the intercourse destitute. Whether you had surgery, you hate being touched down there, or it's just not your day, oral sex can be your friend.

How bad can it be? It won't make you fat. Like celery and grapefruit, it's negative calories. It will help soothe a relationship that needs more than you can deliver. Look at it as a gift. Share sex like you'd share a special dinner: You can choose your entree, but you have to agree on a time and place.

A few technicalities:

• Soap is cheap. Skin folds are tricky. Wash them twice.

• Dentures: Remove them if they don't fit well.

• Breathing is a challenge. If you're oxygen-dependent, secure your oxygen first!

• Sex is exercise. Getting in shape will improve your health, your endurance, and your fun.

• Use condoms if it's just a random night. HIV, HSV, HCV, and gonorrhea don't care about age.

• It's not kosher. I checked.

Still, oral sex may not be your thing, whether you're not that adventurous, you have a gag reflex, or your morals don't agree.

Modern technology is there for you. You can cater to each other's needs without the physical demands. Vibrators conquer challenges that hypertension, diabetes, and strokes make unmanageable. Electricity is cheap.

Caveats:

1. Be careful with batteries. They'll spoil the mood if they catch fire.

2. Avoid vacuum cleaners. They have way too much suction.

3. Avoid vegetables, even healthy ones. They go bad if they break inside.

4. Same with glass. Stick with plastic.

Bottom line: Sex in the elderly is not for the faint of heart, but its a way to stay together even as everything else falls apart: joints, friendships, retirement accounts.

Sex is just another way to love each other and meet each others' needs. Getting them what they need, whether you need it or not, is like you'd get them their cereal even if you live gluten-free.

Sex in the elderly is both a challenge and an opportunity. Like walking with a walker, it's clumsy, but it gets you there.

Until the stairs.

Initially published 12 May 2019 ©RadaJonesMD

40 PRO TIPS FOR YOUR LOVED ONE'S ER VISIT

The ER is stressful. Stressful for the patients, the families, and even the staff. People are sick. Some are dying - some just think they are. The place is chaotic, noisy, and frightening. You'll feel like you've been sitting in the waiting room forever, even if it's only been an hour. Then they'll bring you in, and you'll wait some more. You'll see people who came after your loved one get seen before them. As time drags, your nerves fray and your patience runs out. You want to help your loved one, but you don't know how.

I'll give you some tips that will make your time go faster, and your visit go smoother. They may even help save a life.

1. **Tell us about your loved one.** What brings them in? What's their baseline? What changed today? But don't speak FOR them, unless they can't. That gets us

worried, since that's what abusers often do.

2. **Talk to us about their code status** (what should we do if things turn bad?) and leave us a phone number to contact you if you leave.

3. **Pay attention to them while you're waiting**, and call us if something changes – if they get worse, if they can't talk, if they turn blue. Call us. Not 911. The nurse call button.

4. **Be kind and supportive**. Don't rehash what they should have done. This is not the time. "That's exactly what you deserve, you moron," won't help them, even if it happens to be true.

5. **Don't feed them.** They won't starve in an hour, but feeding them may delay lifesaving procedures like surgery, or endoscopy. That last burger may just be their last.

6. **Don't picnic in the treatment room**. Please step out if you need to eat. Your loved one won't steal your food, and the staff won't keel over because of the smell. They're always hungry, since they seldom get to eat.

7. **Bring in their medications,** their allergies, and their doctor's phone number. You'll get brownie points, and we won't give them the stuff they're allergic to. Plus, we'll do our best to contact their doctor. Win-win.

Stay Away from MY ER and Other Fun Bits ... 73

8. **Bring something to do:** A book, your knitting, an Ipad. Expect to be there for hours. In the ER, things take time.
9. **Don't stand in the door** to give us dirty looks. That won't make us work any faster. If you have to wait, that's good news. In the ER you don't want to go first. The first ones are always the ones fixing to die.
10. **Don't let them pee** without telling us. In the ER, urine is as rare as gold. We need it. If we miss it, that may mean waiting a couple more hours for the next one. You don't want that.
11. **Don't make love in the treatment rooms.** Not even oral sex. It's awkward for the neighbors and it will put you last to be seen. Those who are dying don't have sex. Those having sex aren't dying. Unless they're doing it while driving.
12. **Don't circle your loved one to keep us away.** To care for them, we need to be able to see, hear and touch them. If you don't want us touching them, try telemedicine
13. **Don't interrupt our care to chat to them** or other visitors. Let us do our job first. *"Oh, Margery, how good of you to come! How's the kids? Good! We've been here for hours. He's hurting – aren't you Jo? How's your aunt's dog? I saw him on Facebook. Not your aunt's? Her neighbor's?"* All that while we're trying to speak to the patient and examine them, but we

can't. Remember it's a treatment room, not a cocktail party.

14. **In the ER, VIPs fare poorly.** Asking: "You know who I am?" won't buy you special treatment (unlike our usual crappy one.) Unless you're here often, and then your special treatment may be a care plan. Few patients like them.
15. **Don't take away your loved one's glasses and hearing aids**. I know they're expensive and they may get lost. Remember that your loved one needs to communicate. Taking away their ability to see and hear is like blindfolding them, then sending them to a scary place.
16. **Ditto for dentures**. We promise we won't steal them, even if they look real.
17. **Bring them something nice** when you come to see them: a book, a picture of the cat, a letter from the kids.
18. **Don't bring them alcohol or drugs**, even if they ask. If that's what they need, they'd be better off at the bar down the road.
19. **Ditto for cigarettes, lighters, guns, knives and razor blades**.
20. **Don't make a point of taking notes, unless you tell us why you need them.** That generates hostility. Why document for trial before badness even happened?
21. **Don't record us during procedures to put us on Social Media,** even if you love Dr. Pimple Popper. Our makeup is never on point and we don't get Hollywood pay.

22. **Advocate for your loved ones,** but don't tell us what your aunt's hairdresser said we should do, unless they are moonlighting from their doctor job. Same with Dr. Google. We're all familiar with Google and Facebook. We've even had a little training beyond that.
23. **Don't get touchy-feely with us**. We don't look for dates at work. That's what Tinder is for. Plus, those stains on our scrubs? They're probably not coffee. Keep your hands to yourself.
24. **Please talk to your family.** We'll be happy to talk to an extra person or two – their mother, the nurse, the POA. Not to all 12 siblings, even if they're lovely people – unless they happen to all be there at the same time.
25. **In the ER, whenever you say: "He has a high pain tolerance" we hear: "He has a high tolerance for pain meds."**
26. **Don't threaten us. It won't get you what you want** unless what you want is a Security escort. Talking about lawyers won't help either.
27. **Don't key our cars. Don't slash our tires.** Security cameras are everywhere. It won't feel good for long.
28. **Try to go along with your loved one's choices.** If they like flowers, bring them flowers. If they like Sudoku, bring them Sudoku. If they want to be DNR, let them be DNR.

29. **Don't lie to them-unless they want you to**. We all deserve the truth if we can handle it.
30. **Don't give them their home meds without talking to us first.** Their home meds may make them worse. They may even be why they're sick, like if they took too much insulin, or took too much of their blood pressure medications.
31. **Please don't wait until you get the discharge papers to bring up new issues** – like yesterday's chest pain. That will keep you in the ER even longer.
32. **Take notes of the doctor's explanation, discharge instructions, follow up.** Ask for permission to record it for your loved one to revisit later.
33. **Feel free to ask about our credentials.** We love to brag.
34. **Not all males are doctors. Not all doctors are male. Not all females are nurses.**
35. **Let us know if you're a health care professional, but if you introduce yourself as a doctor, please be aware: In the ER, the only real doctor is a medical doctor.**
36. **Most patients worry more about their kids, pets or spouses than about themselves.** Who'll take Joey off the bus? Who'll let Trixie out? Who'll get Hubs' dinner? Help them plan so they can stay to complete their workup.
37. **Don't bring immunocompromised people, infants, or anyone who doesn't**

need to be here. The ER is Germs Swing Disco. Most patients who come there are sick. Don't expose your newborn, your pregnant wife or your mom who's on chemo to never-ending badness.

38. **Limit the number of visitors**. Patients in crowded rooms get worse care. They can't rest. Performing a rectal exam or getting a urine sample is like relaxing in Walmart – desirable, but unlikely.
39. **When they're done, get them out of here ASAP**. In the ER, every moment is fraught with peril. Every sneeze can be the flu. Every handshake can get them sick. Take them home.
40. **Bring them back if they get worse,** if they don't get better, if you can't follow up as directed. We'd rather correct our mistakes than bury them.

Wishing your loved one a speedy recovery and hoping your visit goes well.

Originally published 21 April 2019 ©RadaJonesMD

CRAZY!

"I can't pee," he says.

"How come?"

"They froze my urethra! They got mad that I didn't listen to them. To punish me, they froze my urethra. Now I can't pee."

"Who froze it?"

"The voices."

The voices froze his urethra.

He's a good-looking man, with his tan setting off his silver buzz cut and nonblinking eyes. He's wearing blue paper scrubs, our mandatory mental health outfit, and he's wearing them well.

The blues help, even though many hate them. They remove the risk of hidden weapons that could harm them or others. They prevent them from overdosing on the pills stashed in their underwear. They set them apart from the other patients, those who can come and go as they please. Blue patients only get bathroom privileges. Plus, the paper is too flimsy to hang yourself with and it saves on laundry.

He smiles. I smile back. I like it better than being cursed, punched and spat at, as usual. I probe further.

"How did they freeze it?"

"By remote control. They put in a chip."

How I wish I had that technology! It would work wonders. No more adult diapers. No more Foleys. It would even help heal decubitus wounds. What a dream!

I sigh. I get back to here and now. It's time to ask the question. The danger question.

"Have you had any thoughts about hurting yourself or others?"

"No. Not me. The wolf-pack."

"The wolf-pack?"

"They told me to kill myself. I didn't. That's why they froze my urethra."

Sometimes it's the FBI, sometimes it's Jesus, sometimes it's the devil. Today it's the wolf-pack.

I'm working a blue shift today. I get my usual share of heart attacks, STDs, and diarrheas, but I'm also in charge of half a dozen or so mental health patients. They're all waiting. For medical clearance, mental health evaluation, a psychiatric bed, a safe place to go.

In my ER, we have three "mental health safe" rooms, stripped of everything but the stretcher. That's seldom enough, so many blue patients lay in the hallways in plain sight. They sleep, they eat, they get bored, they watch the action. Until they become the action.

Some are sick, like Mr. Wolf-Pack. Psychotic, manic, catatonic, despondent. Like Cat-Woman.

She thinks she's a cat. She won't talk. She refuses to eat anything but cat food, and there's no cat food in the cafeteria. I tried milk. She hissed at me.

Some metabolize yesterday's liquor - they got drunk and got into a fight. They said they'll kill themselves, so somebody called 911, and they're here, waiting for a mental health evaluation.

Kids out of control, some as young as five. They had a temper tantrum, so their adults called police to bring them over. They hope for a magic potion to make them into little angels. But since we're not Hogwarts, that doesn't happen. That's why twelve-year-old Johnny, who has developmental delays and autism, has been with us in the ED for 23 days. There's nowhere else for him to go. He eats, he sleeps, he plays cards with the staff. Until he gets angry, rips his blues, and throws feces at us.

Some are demented. The nursing home sent them here because they bit their nurse or they peed in the sink. They didn't know she was their nurse, and to them, the sink looks just like a urinal. They don't know where they are, nor why they're here. Neither do I.

Some suffer from debilitating chronic pain, and they can no longer stand the suffering. They'll kill themselves if I don't give them Dilaudid or Xanax. Preferably both.

Some feel unloved, and they need attention. They took a double dose of Motrin, tried to strangle themselves with their bare hands, or scratched their wrist with a paperclip.

Some are lonely and hopeless. Their wife of fifty years died; the dog, their only friend, got run over by a car; the kids never call.

They all wait for hours, days, weeks, in the ED

purgatory. They get bored watching the walls. They get needy. They need nicotine patches, sandwiches, a third warm blanket, a fifth cup of coffee — not decaf — with four sugars and milk. They need things we can't provide.

They swallow curtain rings and forks to buy themselves an endoscopy, and the sedation that goes with it. They punch the walls or eat paint. They try to elope; they fight. For their safety and ours, we need to sedate and restrain them.

They need love. They flirt with the other blue patients. They get attached to the staff, who go home after their shift, making them feel rejected. They wait. They wait for a long time.

The lucky ones go home. Some will come back tomorrow, and the day after that, and the day after that.

Some get admitted. Some return the day after they get discharged. Some have nowhere to go. The prevalence of mental health illness in the US is staggering, and mental health treatment is elusive. Find out more on RadaJonesMD.com/crazy.

American mental health care is in crisis. The mentally ill suffer. So do their families. So does my ED, choking under the burden of psychiatric patients with no place to go. Mental health illness affects us all. Mr. Wolfpack, Cat-woman, and Johnny need help. Helping them will make us a better society and a better country. We must find resources to help our vulnerable, our endangered, our needy. Helping them will help us all.

If you need help now:

NIMH: If you are in crisis, and need immediate support or intervention, call or go to the website of the National Suicide Prevention Lifeline (1-800-273-8255).

Trained crisis workers are available to talk 24 hours a day, 7 days a week. Your call goes to the nearest crisis center in the Lifeline national network. These centers provide crisis counseling and mental health referrals. If the situation is potentially life-threatening, call 911 or go to a hospital emergency room.

Initially published 9 June 2019 ©RadaJonesMD

TWENTY-FOUR REASONS TO NOT VACCINATE YOUR KID

1. **You don't like to be told what to do.** Especially not by arrogant doctors, who act as if they know better, just because they've been through a few decades of training!
2. **Your child hates shots.** And, as her parent, your feel that your main job is to keep her comfortable rather than safe.
3. **You're more worried about side effects and complications than you are about tetanus and meningitis.** You heard about the two deaths from vaccination errors in Samoa, but not about the 83 Measles deaths. Because you don't trust the media. *"The pro-vaccine mafia is quick to sweep all cases of vaccine-related injury and death under the rug as extremely rare anomalies, but many a parent of a vaccine-injured child will be the first to tell you that, if she could do it all over again, she wouldn't*

have let her kid get jabbed," the anti-vaxxers say.

4. You once got the flu after you got the flu vaccine, so you know that **vaccines don't work.** Newsflash: they do. Just not 100%. Nothing works 100%
5. **You read somewhere that vaccines weaken immunity.** Tetyana Obukhanych Ph.D. states: *"in the debate over vaccine safety, we have lost sight of a bigger problem: how vaccination campaigns wipe out our herd immunity and endanger the very young."* You didn't notice the disclaimer: *"The information in this book is not intended as medical advice. Readers assume sole responsibility for choosing for themselves and their children disease prevention options that are compatible with their convictions."* No medical advice here. How about getting some medical advice from your kid's doctor?
6. **Taking your kid to the doctor takes time.** Plus, doctors are always late, like they're taking care of sick kids or something, and you don't have time for this.
7. **Vaccines cost money.** Not yours, of course, they come from the insurance. But you still have to pay for the gas.
8. Jenny McCarthy and other celebrities, including a famous – now infamous – doctor, whose license was withdrawn for fraud, say that **vaccines can lead to autism**. The entire medical community

disagrees, but you trust Jenny more than you trust your pediatrician.
9. **You think that your pediatrician is looking to make money** out of your child. After all, pediatricians are well known to be rich.
10. **You can't sue the vaccine companies** if your child is harmed. The National Childhood Vaccine Injury Act of 1986 exempts drug companies from liability, in an effort to avoid vaccine shortage. But did you know that that law establishes alternative ways to compensate those who have been harmed?
11. You read that "**vaccines can cause lifelong, incurable diseases**… if your child develops permanent nerve damage, she could require lifelong care… If you choose to vaccinate, are you prepared to reorient your life in the event of autism or brain damage?" So, you'd rather let them take their chance with childhood diseases. Are you familiar with Polio and its damaging long-term consequences?
12. **You always wanted a boy**. This one is a girl.
13. **Vaccines kill children**. Your anti-vaxx resources told you that "Gardasil, the HPV vaccine, has injured and killed tens of thousands of adolescents and teenagers." While you're looking for the mass graves, how about checking what CDC has to say?

14. **You know better than anyone what's best for your child**, so you don't need to take her to a doctor. She shares your DNA. You don't need an education or even information. It's all in your DNA.
15. **Even Gandhi was against vaccines**. For him, it wasn't really about vaccines. It was about cows. He disapproved of using cows to produce the smallpox vaccine. He also disapproved of eating them. He didn't do steaks, not even burgers. He was a Hindu and a fruitarian. Are you?
16. **Vaccines contain toxic stuff**. As a matter of fact, vaccines are mostly water and antigen, plus preservatives to keep them from going bad. Because you wouldn't inject rotten stuff into your kids, would you? Those preservatives are similar to those in your packaged bread, soda, mayo, and mascara. Are you foregoing all those?
17. **Your kid looks like your ex.** And you hate your ex.
18. **Vaccines will overwhelm your baby's immune system**. Newsflash: Your baby doesn't have an immune system. Yet. That's what vaccines are doing. Building up her immune system to help her fight disease.
19. **The immunocompromised who can't be immunized and are at risk – young babies, cancer kids, pregnant women – they're not your problem.** They'd better take care of themselves.

20. **Childhood diseases have been mostly eradicated. Why vaccinate for something that doesn't even exist?** Good point! That's why we no longer vaccinate for smallpox. Because it's extinct. Why? Because of the vaccine. We vaccinate for other diseases. Measles, mumps, pertussis. They've been resurging since people stopped vaccinating. Google Samoa's measles outbreak, its cause and its consequences.

21. **God says NO**. Like some in the Middle East, you think that vaccinating your kids is against God's will. Many loving parents in Pakistan and Afghanistan thought that the Polio vaccine was intended to prevent their kids from reproducing. Not really. The vaccine was meant to prevent the kids from getting paralyzed by Polio. Still, angry mobs killed healthcare workers to fulfill God's wish. I don't think that really helped their children.

22. **You heard that natural exposure to disease is better than vaccines.** *"Truth be told, the only way to truly develop vibrant, lifelong immunity, is to live your life as you normally would, without injecting dead viruses and chemical adjuvants into your muscle tissue. Natural exposure to whatever diseases are lurking in the world is the only way for the body to develop permanent antibodies that will forever protect against disease."* There's some truth to that. The immunity they will get after having a

disease is likely to be stronger than that obtained from vaccines. Presuming that they survive the disease. Some won't. Are you willing to take that risk?
23. **Unlike the others, your child is special**. Believe it or not, but most parents feel that way. Their kids are special to them.
24. **The earth is overpopulated** anyhow.

I'll offer you a compromise: **Don't vaccinate all your kids. Only vaccinate the ones you want to keep.**

For those who can't immunize your kids for medical reasons: take care and stay safe!

Originally published 9 Feb 2019 ©RadaJonesMD

WHY DOCTORS MAKE BAD PATIENTS

I'm a doctor. And, like most medical professionals, I'm a terrible patient.

Two years after my last appointment, I got a CTJ, "Come to Jesus" from my doctor. I had called his office since I needed a form stating that I don't have tertiary syphilis for my Thai visa. Why tertiary syphilis, as opposed to Ebola, HIV, cholera, lepers, or bubonic plague? I don't know. That's the power of bureaucracies. They don't have to make sense. They get to make the rules.

My doctor wasn't happy. "Come get seen or get lost," he said. Or something to that effect, politely wrapped.

I went.

Good news: I didn't have tertiary syphilis.

Bad news: I didn't have a colonoscopy either. At 57, I'm seven years late. I didn't have a recent mammogram either. As for the PAP smear...

Whatever you think, I'm not totally negligent. I brush my teeth. I floss. I pay attention to what I eat. Too much, maybe. I work out. I don't smoke. Anything.

But I live and work in a small community in the North Country. I know every doctor, including the vets. I work daily with the OBGYNs and the GIs. Nice people. Down to earth, outdoorsy, mostly easy-going. I love seeing them in the ER, though they seldom feel the same way. We commiserate about the weather, we bash the administrators' latest move, we're friends on Facebook. I know the names of their dogs, the size of their wives, and how many cocktails they've had before posting on Facebook.

I like them, but a colonoscopy? That's a level of carnal knowledge I'm not up for.

I don't know about you, but I find it easier to show my privates to people I don't know than to my friends. Having them examine my insides – and my outsides – is not my idea of fun. Not like it's life and death, people! Yes, I see them in the ER. I even intubated a few. But they didn't have a choice! They were dying!

My doctor got it. He didn't care.

"You need preventive care. You're way past due for colon cancer screening. And pap smear."

"But I've never had a bad pap smear! And my social life is not worth mentioning!"

He nodded, smiled, and referred me across the lake, in the next state, for GYN. He got me Cologard.

What's Cologard? It's a test for colon cancer that doesn't require a colonoscopy. You provide a sample (of you know what) in the comfort of your own home, then send it for DNA testing.

I can do that, I thought.

Stay Away from MY ER and Other Fun Bits ...

Yesterday was Christmas in July. The mailman brought me a Doximity plaque proclaiming me "The most entertaining author," and a cardboard box of Cologard with multiple interrelated plastic parts and 80 pages of bilingual instructions.

Did you ever buy furniture from Ikea? It's DIY, and it comes in boxes. The instructions are more entertaining than straightforward. My success rate is 1:3 - three assemblies to get one right. Cologard must use the same writers.

Instructions started with Step 6: Label your samples.

That's jumping the gun a little, I thought. But I didn't let that deter me.

Next brochure: How to return your kit. Four pages later, I got enlightened: Weekend pooping is a no-no. The package needs to be sent immediately and tested within 48 hours.

Further explorations brought me to another unputdownable 60-page brochure. Indications, contraindications, warning, precautions, test interpretation, risks, and more. The style was crisp, the images graphic, the protagonist daring.

Twelve pages into it, I got to Step 1: Check the expiration date, then to Step 2: Prepare to collect a stool sample. How to assemble your Cologard kit and avoid pooping next to it. Or something to that effect.

I pulled the heavy zipper bag out of the box to remove the contents. It wouldn't come. I pulled harder. Nope. I turned it upside down and shook it. It was stuck.

I tore it off the box. Then I saw it, right there. Leave the plastic bag and the white tray inside the box.

I pushed it back to cover the tear, and I engrossed myself in the lecture. Half an hour later, I'm an expert in Cologard. I can't wait to test my new expertise once the weekend is over.

The pap-smear, you say? Seriously? I hope he forgets about it!

But that got me thinking. Am I foolish to avoid preventive care? I wouldn't let my patients do that. Am I risking my health? My life maybe? Why?

Is it because I'm a doctor? Do I secretly believe that my medical knowledge will keep me safe? That I'll know it if my body goes rogue?

Or is it just the opposite? Do I know enough about medicine, including how little we really know, to lose respect for the science?

There's so much we don't know. Then, half of what we do know is wrong. We just don't know which half. From blood-letting to smoking and coffee, the only constant in medicine is change. This here is just the latest.

Or is it the NNS, the number needed to screen, that makes me fatalistic? 25,000 to prevent one death from melanoma. 1374 (every five years) for colon cancer, 2451 for mammograms. They cost money and time. They have risks. Many risks. False positives, exposing you to more studies. Colon perforation. Infection. Bleeding. Sedation gone bad. More.

Is that why I'm a lousy patient? Maybe. But I'm not an exception. Most medical professionals are the same.

We all should take better care of ourselves. We all should sleep more, drink less, avoid stress, get our colonoscopies, and our mammograms. Ask for help when we need it. We'd live better and longer.

But we don't. Why?

I hope I remember that next time I get upset with my patients for being noncompliant.

In the meantime, I'll go look for some essential oils. Anybody knows how to grow aloe?

Initially published 3 Aug 2019 ©RadaJonesMD

WHAT'S SO HARD ABOUT THE ER?

I work in the ER. It's not an easy job. Not glamorous either. At least not as exciting as my Mother-in-Law used to think.

Years ago, when I declared I was going into Emergency, she looked at me askance. She didn't ask me why. She just looked at me with her wise old eyes. "Let me tell you about ER," she said. "I know all about it. I watched every show."

She was politely dismissive and actively unimpressed. Worried about her daughter-in-law having sex in the closets, maybe? She thought that my hair and my style won't stand up to the job?

She was right. Not about sex. I don't know how the folks in the movies find the time. Or the interest. I struggle to find time to pee. And the closets? Really? You get turned on by dirty mops and bleach perfume? She was right about the hair. It's still not worth mentioning. And my style – what style?

I eventually got used to people questioning my

career choice. Patients ask me when I'm going to specialize. My best friend – a computer maven – asked me why I choose to work triage. "Can't a nurse do that? Shouldn't you be treating people instead?" I tried to explain. She smiled and changed the subject. I got even by questioning her choice of husbands. Years later, we're still friends. She dispoed her husband, but I still work in the ER. Advantage home.

Still, every once in a while, somebody asks me a question that catches me off-guard. **"What's the hardest thing about your job?"**

I stumble. I mumble. I try to say something intelligent. I fail. They try to help.

"Is it people dying?" they ask.

No, it's not, even though I feel defeated every time someone dies on my watch. Even if there was nothing I could do. I feel inadequate and powerless. I always wonder if a smarter doctor, a faster doctor, a better doctor, could save them. I agonize about it, looking for my failing. But that's not the hardest part of my job.

"Is it the abuse? Is it people swearing at you, throwing feces at you, keying your car, and threatening to rape your daughter?"

I don't have a daughter. I don't even own a car. And, after all these years, I got used to the swearing and being called the c-word. I don't like the feces or the spit, nor being bitten or kicked, but I use protective equipment, and I do my best to stay out of the fray. And, when everything else fails, IM SUX works. I've yet to see somebody spitting with a plastic tube in their throat.

"Is it your accent? These days, immigration has become a dirty word."

No. People spend their last hard-fought breath to find out where I'm from. Romania, I used to say. That was the end of the conversation. Awkward. I stopped telling them. If they insist, I say Beekmantown. My nurses love it. They can't wait to get in on the game. If I say Transylvania, patients think I'm kidding. We laugh and get back to what matters – what they're there for. Once only, my Dilaudid-deficient patient asked for an English-speaking doctor. I think she meant American. My English isn't that bad.

"Is it telling families that their loved one died?"

No. It's never easy, even if they lived to be a hundred, but it's part of the job. I try to make it easy on them. I wash my hands of their loved one's blood. I borrow a clean coat, even if I have to cover somebody else's name with my badge. I lie. I pretend it didn't hurt them, and it didn't hurt me. I do my best to give them solace.

"Is it being a woman? Having to deal with the glass ceiling?"

Not really, though it's still frustrating when patients call you "Nurse!" after introducing yourself as their doctor. I didn't suffer much from the glass ceiling. I didn't aim high enough? A perk of age? By the time I got to be a doctor, I was past maternity leave. And I found handling angry surgeons easier than dealing with macho men in Communist Romania.

"Is it the human tragedy? The drunk drivers, the sexual assaults, the children with broken bones and cigarette burns on their belly? Is this the hardest part?"

No. These are all things I can do something

about. I treat, I advocate, I educate. I struggle to prevent it from happening. I try to make a difference.

"What is it, then?" they ask.

It's making decisions. Choosing winners and losers, when I don't know who should win and who should lose. Every shift I make decisions with limited information, limited resources and limited time. Decisions that can mean somebody's life or death.

Some are big: Do I scan this back pain, looking for a dissection, and possibly destroy his kidneys, or do I send him home to maybe die.

Some are small: Should I first discharge Room 9, who's desperate to get her kids off the bus, or see the chest pain in Room 3, which may be having a heart attack?

Some, I don't even know. This woman, here for the third time this week, is she a drug seeker? Or is she sick? Should I scan her again, spending thousands of dollars on her third workup? Or should I have security escort her out?

This smiling infant with a bruise on her neck. Is she an adventurous explorer, or an abused child that I'm about to send home to die? Should I call CPS and destroy the peace of this family, or should I trust her sobbing mother telling me she stumbled and fell on a toy?

And of course, they all come at the same time: the chest pain, the baby, the fire drill, the EMS call, the floor code, the radiologist calling about the brain bleed, the administrator barking at me for being behind on my charts.

I can't do it all. Not at the same time. But maybe

a smarter doctor, a faster doctor, a better doctor, she could.

The hardest part of my job is the guilt. I never, ever, do everything I should. Not well enough, not fast enough, and never perfect.

First published on Doximity.com on 29 Aug 2019, as "What's The Hardest Part of Practicing Emergency Medicine?" ©RadaJonesMD

STRANGEST REAL PATIENT COMPLAINTS, PART 3

1. Patient in the ER for vulvar pain: "My labia got tangled in my underwear." It required a procedure to set it free.

2. Triage note: "Patient states that she got hit in the head with a frozen burrito that flew off the assembly line."

3. Patient's boyfriend call to EMS: "Her cummer is stuck." The patient had a seizure during sex.

4. "My acid reflux came out my ears after I ate."

5. 911 call: "I need an ambulance. I dropped a jar of peanut butter on my toe, and I think it's bruised."

6. "I have sperm dripping from my vagina."

7. Triage note: "Patient comes for knee pain and bruising. He states that he fell as he was running from an ostrich."

8. Contrite elderly patient: "I swallowed my wife's hearing aids."

9. Triage note: "The family states that a live bat

was found in their attic. Didn't hit anyone or bite them, but the whole family of 6, including those who were not home, insists on getting rabies IgG."

10. "I kissed a girl, not my girlfriend, and now my cum tastes different."

11. "I'm bleeding from my mouth after oral sex."

12. Triage note: "The patient comes for a fractured penis. His 300 lbs partner was on top, and she bounced the wrong way."

13. "I got raped by my dildo."

14. Male patient who googled his symptoms: "I think I have ovarian cancer."

15. Triage note: "The patient injected his testicles with industrial-grade silicone with a manual bicycle tire pump,"

16. "I have an enlarged Prostrate.

17. Triage note: "Patient drove himself to the ER after being gored by a buffalo. He was loading his herd onto a truck, and they stampeded. He drove himself in with significant injuries."

18. "I have a pinched nerve right above my testicles."

19. Triage note: "The patient complains of anxiety brought on by two days in a silent retreat. She states it was too quiet."

20. "I have a pussy discharge."

21. EMS report: "The patient states he stuck a bottle of cocoa butter lotion in his colon to get out of jail, and now he can't get it out."

22. "I was playing with magnets. They stuck together, and I can't get them off my junk."

23. Elderly smoker: "I've had trouble breathing since birth."

24. EMS call: "The patient states he got his nuts stuck in a lawn chair."

25. Triage note: "Patient states her iguana took off half her finger."

26. "I pulled a worm off my butt."

27. Trauma code: 68 years old female scalped by her horse, who bit off her hair bun.

28. "I ate the wrong vagina."

29. Triage note: "Patient states she is here for possible inhalation of potato chips."

30. "I'm pretty sure I'm a dead man walking."

31. Triage note: "Patient states he got into a fight with a raccoon."

32. Patient staring at the doctor: "I'm starting to see Satan."

33. Triage note: "The patient fell on an 8lb sledgehammer that got stuck in his butt, then drove himself to the ER."

34. "I got run over by a pig." Patient works at a slaughterhouse and got trampled by a 350 lb pig.

35. EMS report: "The patient's girlfriend shoved a knife up his rectum, blade first, as he was tied to the bed." He got a colostomy.

36. "I think I broke my penis. It's crooked."

37. Nursing home patient brought in for altered mental status: "They say I have smoke in my attic!"

38. Elderly patient with conjunctivitis: "A squirrel urinated in my eye."

39. Fast-track patient with eye pain: "A baby turkey pecked me in the corner of my eye."

40. Triage note: "Patient states her legs are turning blue." It was dye from her new jeans.

41. "I got monkey poo in my face, and I'm worried I got HIV."

42. Triage note: "The patient complains of getting bit by a zebra."

43. "I have a dead kitten hanging from my lip." She kissed it, it bit her, she choked it.

44. "I ate sushi two years ago. Now there's a parasite crawling out of my skin."

45. Self-triage form filled by a patient: "I got apesex and pain." Not the right way to spell abscess.

46. EMS call: "The patient requests transport to ED for Valtrex. His girlfriend told him she had herpes. The second unit is bringing her. She has been assaulted."

47. "I went to take a shower. My wife had put a zucchini on the bathroom chair. I sat down to dry my feet."

48. "I've been sick for twenty years, but I'm worse tonight."

Lessons learned:

1. Avoid animals and birds from ostriches to zebras. Even pussies.

2. Sex is risky. Always play is safe.

3. With a name like Smucker's, it's got to be good.

Thanks to my many ER friends who contributed to this list.

Initially published 4 Feb 2019 ©RadaJonesMD

OBAMACARE VS. UNIVERSAL HEALTHCARE

I'll start with a shameful confession: I hated Obamacare. The day it passed, I was so angry that I stopped talking to my husband. It wasn't his fault they did it, but he was an ardent supporter, while I thought it to be the most ill-conceived piece of legislation ever.

I was right.

Obama care was a patch to a national health system crumbling under its own weight. It had thousands and thousands of pages, but no rhyme or reason. Have you seen "The Money Pit?" You put in a little money. You put a little more. You fix this glitch. That creates another, leading to a loophole that the shrewd take advantage of. The others? They crumble under the weight of unfunded mandates.

The good news? We created more and more well-paid jobs. We got more regulators to implement more metrics in the elusive hope to cut costs.

They didn't recoup the money their jobs cost. The healthcare costs went through the roof. So what? We'll just cut some nurses.

In the meantime, we'll employ more administrators, buy more computers, get more EHRs. We need them to count the exact number of days a patient has to stay in the hospital before he can go to a nursing home.

His doctor knows, his family knows, his cat knows. He doesn't need the hospital. He needs long term care.

Not so fast! Criteria established by people who've never touched a patient say otherwise. He needs an ER visit and at least three nights before long term care. And you wonder where the money goes?

Obamacare expanded Medicare and Medicaid. I wish that would help my patients.

In my community ER, neither my patients nor I saw a neurologist for years. We used to have one, but she went bankrupt and moved to Maine. Our urologists – the few still left - don't take Medicaid, since the pay doesn't even cover the office cleaning. Our last ENT retired at 90. Our dermatologist has a six-month wait. It's the same with GI and Orthopedics.

Let's be clear: health insurance and health care are not the same thing. Giving my patients Medicaid is pretty much like giving them Monopoly money. They may be able to get St. James' Place, but not lithotripsy. And, as more and more criteria bog down Medicare, fewer doctors accept patients who don't help their bottom line.

Bad doctors! Greedy doctors, you say. Not mine. Where I come from, doctors wear jeans instead of suits and drive Subarus and Chevys instead of German cars. There's not a single BMW or Mercedes dealer in my hometown.

But I digress. We were talking about Obamacare. Making more rules created by non-clinicians to regulate clinical work to improve compliance. More paper-pushers draining the hospital budget to monitor care. That's OK. We'll just cut down on nursing jobs. Safe staffing, anyone?

Implementing Obamacare was like putting new tires on your 250K Chevy truck. It'll help until the breaks fail or the engine falls off. Like painting the walls without fixing the roof. But even more importantly, Obamacare is not universal healthcare, like most civilized nations have.

Even communist Romania had it. We didn't have enough to eat, but I had a doctor. So did my mother, my grandmother and everybody else I knew. I got free vaccines and free medications. I had never heard about not having a doctor or a dentist. I never went to the ER. When I got sick, I saw my doctor. I saw her even when I wasn't sick for my yearly check-up.

Not here. In the wealthiest, most powerful country in the world, our life expectancy is falling. What's life expectancy? For the simple-minded, like me, it's how long a kid born today is likely to live. The longer, the better.

In 2016, the WHO put the USA at #31 in the world in life expectancy, sandwiched between Costa Rica and Cuba, behind Chile, Slovenia, Greece, and Cyprus.

The 2018 CIA World Factbook puts us at #45. We're behind Turks and Caicos but ahead of Wallis and Futuna. What's Wallis and Futuna, you ask?

"The Futuna island group was discovered by the Dutch in 1616 and Wallis by the British in 1767, but it was the French who declared a protectorate over the islands in 1842…In 2003, Wallis and Futuna's designation changed to that of an overseas collectivity."

I now realize that my paranoid patient in Room 6 was right. CIA does know everything. They must have cameras in his pills like he said.

So: The good news: we're doing better than Wallis and Futuna.

The bad news: our ranking is falling. We expect to be #61 in 2040, when Spain will reach #1, overtaking Japan. It's got to be either the shorter work hours, or Rioja's health benefits compared to Sake.

As per CDC "(USA)…life expectancy at birth decreased for the second consecutive year in 2016, mainly due to increases in mortality from unintentional injuries, homicide, Alzheimer's disease, suicide, and Parkinson's disease." This is not good news.

The main reason I hated Obamacare was politics. I felt that once politicians got to brag about providing health insurance, there would be no incentive to fight for real health reform. I believed that Obamacare took the option of universal healthcare off the table. That lost opportunity will haunt us for generations. And I think I was right.

The fight around Obamacare and healthcare reform is about to shape the 2020 elections – for the good or the bad. Regardless of who wins and who loses, my wish for 2020 is that one way or another, my patients will get the healthcare they need. I want every kid to have a doctor, every pregnant woman to get prenatal care, and every man to see a dentist - at least twice a year.

And I really hope we don't fall behind Wallis and Futuna, even though I wish them only the best.

Initially published 31 March 2019 ©Rada Jones MD

PATIENTS SAY THE DARNEDEST THINGS

ER is not an easy place to be for anybody – the patients, their families, and even the staff. The daily dose of suffering and death is emotionally draining. To make it through, you need a thick skin, a sick sense of humor, or both.

Add to that the difficulty of communicating – Medicalese is a language only known to the Medical natives, and English can be the second language for both the staff and the patient . You end up with lousy communication and lots of fun.

The doctor: I'm afraid your ankle is fractured.
Patient: That's it? Thank God it's not broken!

Patient: Nurse, I threw up my IV Toradol.

Doctor: Do you have any medical problems?

Patient: No, but I had Smiling Mighty Jesus when I was a kid. (*Spinal meningitis*)

Doctor: Did you have a CT scan when you were here last?
Patient: No, there was no cat. It was something to do with a puppy. (*Pet scan.*)

Seizure patient: My cat is so smart, she smells my seizures. She learned from the dog... but they aren't talking any more.

Diabetic patient in for hypoglycemia: My sugar isn't high. I know it, since I always taste my pee, so I know when it's too sweet.

Patient to X-ray tech: Don't forget to cover my nuts. And I'll move my phone, so that the X-ray doesn't mess it up.

Patient: I took subliminal nitroglycerin.
Doc, checking the low blood pressure: Good idea!

Patient with a light bulb in his rectum: I was in the shower and I fell on it.

. . .

Seventy years old lost his beer tab pull. **Nurse**: "Where did you lose it?

Patient: "Up my ass."

Wife, calling from home: "You're good, Billy. I found it. It was under the sheets."

Triage nurse: Are you sexually active?

Patient, shaking her head: No, he does most of the work.

Triage sign in sheet: 1. Name. DOB. 3. Sex.

Patient answers: 1. Jenny. 2. March 4th. 3. Five times.

Patient diagnosed with multiple personality disorder: You'd better give me my Ativan right now if you don't want my alternate personality to come out.

Nurse, discharging a patient: Condoms and contraceptive gels, together, are more than 99% effective against pregnancy.

Patient: "I can't do it. I tried the gel on toast. It tastes awful."

Patient brought in for AMS (altered mental status): I'm addicted to meth, women and fried chicken.

. . .

Patient providing his medical history: I have a filter in my Venal Cavern.

Patient's wife: He's got Sea Roaches of the liver. *(cirrhosis)*

Demented patient, looking at a nurse's tattoo: "Cool tattoo! I have one too, you know. It's a mouse on my thigh!" She pulls up her gown to look for it. She looks and looks. "I can't find it. My pussy must have eaten it!"

Nurse: I'm sorry, do you need something?
    Screaming patient, smiling politely: I don't need anything, I'm just crazy.

Blue-haired patient speaking to her young nurse: You know, last night I met a man whose bits still work. And by his bits, I mean his wallet.

Terminally ill patient looking fondly at his lovely nurse: It's got to be good to be a hospice nurse. Everyone's dying to meet you!

Elderly widow who's a stroke patient: Does your wife know that you're spending all this time in my bedroom?

. . .

Elderly patient brought in by ambulance, being undressed by staff: "Ladies, I've only known you for two minutes and you're already taking my clothes off! You guys are fast!"

Lovely elderly patient in the ER for a fever: You know, my grandkids no longer call me grandma. They call me donor!

Middle-aged patient during pelvic exam: Take it easy! I've had five kids, you know. Be careful you don't fall in!

Septic demented patient to the nurse trying to get blood: You just stick me with that needle, and I'll shove it up your ass!

Polite new hospice patient: Where do we go to get killed?

Elderly patient to family: The doctor said he won't cremate me, since I'm not dead yet!

Nurse to diabetic old vet: " I'm going to cover you with insulin."
    Old vet: "Better cover me with your body."

. . .

Night nurse joking as she's giving a patient his vitamins: "Here's your morning Viagra!"

Elderly patient: "Good. That's the only thing that keeps me from rolling out of bed!"

OB nurse, reviewing discharge instructions: "No sex, tampons or douching for six weeks."

Patient, surrounded by her four kids, her parents, and her in-laws: "Will you please repeat that to my husband?"

Patient is covered in blood after pulling out his own IV.

Nurse: "Jesus, you look like you committed a crime!"

Patient, shaking his head: "I'll save that for later!"

Nurse, to the patient exposing himself: "John, I'm sick of seeing your penis!"

Patient, nodding: "Me too!"

Intoxicated pregnant patient positive for meth is offered Tylenol: "Are you sure it's OK for the baby?

Anaphylactic patient: I'm allergic to epinephrine. It makes my heart race.

. . .

Nurse, to septic patient: "I'm sorry, I need to place a Foley catheter in your privates."
Patient shrugs: "Then you'd better make sure to wipe away the cobwebs down there first. It's been a while."

Registration to elderly patient: "Sir, when where you born?"
Patient shrugging: "How the hell do I know? I was too young!"

Patient's son: "Doctor, can you prescribe a pill that would make my Mom happy?"
Doctor, shrugging: "Nope. If I could, I'd be rich!"

Patient's daughter, after being told her mother's gangrenous foot needed amputation: Will her foot grow back?

Night nurse before dawn: "Good morning ma'am, I'm here to get some blood from you."
Patient: "Dracula, you thirsty bitch!"

Mental health patient to counsellor: You know, you really piss me off. But I like you!

. . .

Patient in labor, after pushing for two hours: "I've had it. I don't want to do this any more. I'm going home."

Diabetic patient: Is diabetes contagious? My dog sleeps with me every night!

Patient with flank pain landing over the stretcher: If I pass a kidney stone, will it come out of my clitoris?

Dehydrated patient getting IV fluids: Don't give me that! I'm allergic to normal saline. It always makes me pee.

Mental health practitioner performing a mental health exam: "What month is this?"
    Patient: "Capricorn."

Triage nurse: "Are you thinking about hurting yourself or anybody else?"
    Patient: "Depends on how long the wait is."

Patient: I'm allergic to sodium pentothal. It always makes me go unconscious.

Female patient in the ER for a vaginal discharge: Chlamydia runs in my family!

. . .

Family member: My sister is allergic to Narcan. It makes her freak out.

Triage nurse: "Is there anybody with heart disease in your family?"
    Patient: "Yes. Both my husband and his dad."

Nursing home patient moving around the the meatloaf on her tray: "Is this Gary? The one who died yesterday?"

ER nurse, after placing an IV: "I'll hook you up now."
    Patient: "Please don't! Last time I got hooked up I got syphilis!"

Thanks to my ER friends for contributing to this list.

Initially published 22 Dec 2018 ©Rada Jones MD

THE PILL

"**If you convince people that they're sick, you're in for oodles of money,**" a recent pharmaceutical article said. "They'll come looking for your stuff."

They're wrong. I'm an ER doc, so I know. They'll come anyhow.

They've been coughing for a week, and they can't sleep. Their joints hurt. They get out of breath whenever they take the stairs, and have palpitations every time things don't go their way. Their back's been hurting for ten years. They rolled their ankle three days ago, and it still hurts. Their 92-year-old mother doesn't remember her phone number. Their daughter has belly pain every time she gets her period. They couldn't keep anything down since last January. They googled their itchy navel, and they think it's cancer.

They come to the ER looking for a quick fix for their long-standing symptoms. They bring their anxiety, their pain, their breathlessness, their unrequited wishes. They bring their life – and it's not the one they hoped for. They want it fixed, and they want it NOW.

In our society, we expect immediate gratification. We don't know how to wait, and we don't condone disappointment. Our question needs an instant answer, and our problem needs an instant fix. We Google, instead of going to a library. We text instead of writing a letter. We call in pizza instead of cooking dinner. We order online instead of going shopping. We take digital pictures instead of developing film. We don't even have to go to the movies – they stream to us. Our every wish gets fulfilled in minutes.

Thus primed, we expect the same from our healthcare. There's got to be a pill for it. After all, that's what Big Pharma says: "Take this pill to lose weight. This pill will fix your diabetes. This pill will get rid of your pain, your depression, your constipation, your psoriasis, your incontinence. This pill will make you healthier, more attractive, and will get rid of all your problems.

Oh, boy, do I wish it were so! I'd fix myself first.

My patients come to me to fix their life. I just need to write them a script. Their TV tells them every day:

"Talk to your doctor about X. Ask if X is right for you. There's only one X. Ask for it by name."

They see the ads: Smiling people having fun, playing golf, holding hands with attractive partners while sitting in twin bathtubs watching the ocean. All glowing, ready to have the sex of their lives, as they share their quick fix.

"Millions of people just like you, breathe better/show their cleavage but not their psoriasis/satisfy a hot partner/. Thanks to this pill/powder/patch."

Gazillions of them, all having a great life. Everybody but you. You're at the end of your rope. You need to get the pill that will teleport you into the life you deserve. You need that script, and you need it now. So you come to the ER to get it.

TV ads make today's America look like a nation of bald, fat, impotent, constipated folks with yellow teeth. I hope we are more than that. More than a nation of overfed, depressed, entitled, and desperate pill seekers looking for an instant fix to the problems our excesses have caused. **TV ads tell us that a better life and a better version of ourselves is only a pill away.**

Sadly, it isn't so.

Pills are mostly ineffective, always expensive, often dangerous. You don't think so? Check these excerpts from TV ads, all spoken in a soft, soothing voice (at double speed) while watching happy people frolicking amongst butterflies:

"some people have had changes in behavior, hostility, agitation, depressed mood, and suicidal thoughts or actions while taking or after stopping X..."

"tell your doctor if you experience increased gambling, sexual or other intense urges..."

"May cause you to feel drowsy or fall asleep during normal activities such as driving..."

"May increase the chance of serious skin reactions or stomach and intestine problems such as bleeding or ulcers, which can occur without warning and may cause death..."

"May increase the chance of heart attack or stroke, leading to death..."

My patients come to the ER with their bag-

fulls of drugs. They take them, then they suffer from side effects. So they get more drugs to counteract them. Who benefits from this, you think?

These people are not terminally ill. They're miserable due to their age, bad genes, bad luck, and lack of adequate self-care. That's a hard pill for them to swallow.

I'll go out on a limb and say some truths that need to be told, and I'm sorry if they offend you.

1. **There is yet no pill to make you slim.** You need to move more and eat less. Otherwise, no wealthy person would be fat.

2. **No medicine will stop you from smoking.** Some may help. Most won't. You need to make a plan and follow it. If you fail, try again.

3. **There's no pill to make your life better**. You need to work on it.

4. **No medicine can fix the national epidemic of obesity, diabetes, depression, and desperation that inhabits today's America.**

6. There's no pill to fix the strain of an extra 200 lbs of weight on your knees. No medicine for the damage to your lungs caused by 40 years of smoking. No pill for the deconditioning of 50 years of sedentary living. No tablet for the alienation of living in a nursing home with nobody coming to visit.

7. **There's no pill to fix a broken life, and no pill to fix loneliness.**

8. **The drugs that will help you escape life's misery will get you in trouble.**

If I had a pill to fix any one of those things, I'd be rich. Big Pharma may disagree, but fortunately, they have better things to do than read my rant. Like sell you useless drugs to make money.

Initially published 30 Dec 2018 ©Rada Jones MD.

STAY AWAY FROM MY ER: MORE TIPS

---

1. **Don't put on mascara while you're driving.**
2. **Don't have sex while you're driving either.** It won't feel good for long.
3. We're ER folks. We do emergencies. Our tests look for emergencies. If you come to the ER for anything but an emergency, you're in the wrong place. **Seeing an ER doc for a non-emergent problem is like seeing a cardiologist for your diarrhea**.
4. **Don't leave your meds around for your toddler to sample**. Check grandma's house too.
5. **Fibromyalgia is seldom lethal** for patients, even though it kills me.
6. **Get a doctor**. Your own. He's better than me at managing your blood pressure, your diabetes, your ED (erectile dysfunction). Cheaper too. It will save

you time. You'll have a long wait if you come to the ER for a Viagra script. And I have no free samples.

7. **Help others.** Help your neighbors. Volunteer within your community. Focus less on yourself and more on others. It will make you happier and healthier.
8. **Get rid of your trampoline,** unless you don't really like your kids that much.
9. **Don't hurt my feelings** by telling me that you really, really hate doctors. It won't help our relationship, nor your ER visit.
10. **Overweight is bad**. Bad for your back, bad for your knees, bad for your diabetes. Most of us eat too much and move too little. Next time you're thinking Fudge Sundae, try an apple and a walk instead. I know, walking is for the dogs. Get one. People with pets are healthier, happier and have more fun.
11. **If you're calling the ER to ask how busy we are, you don't need to come.**
12. **Get a dentist**. Teeth are a great investment. They brighten your smile. They make you look younger. They're prettier than tattoos. They can even chew your steak!
13. **Stop smoking!** You won't set your house on fire. You'll save money. Your doctor will stop harassing you. You'll set a good example for your kids. Your car will smell better, and so will you.

14. **Don't lock your children in the car**. Ever. Not in summer, not in winter, not on Wednesdays. Find childcare or take them with you. Same with pets.
15. **Don't fry bacon naked.**
16. **Don't ride your bike while you're walking your dog.**
17. **Don't keep shampoo bottles on the floor.** They tend to get lodged in people's rectums.
18. **Don't keep bleach in soda bottles.** If you do, don't leave them sitting around for your kids to drink them.
19. **Invest in a cock-ring with a release,** and a butt plug with a wide flange. It's cheaper than a trip to the ED. Less embarrassing too.
20. **If you can't control your anger, punch a pillow.** Walls, doors, and windows tend to fight back. Have you heard about Boxer's fractures? They seldom result from boxing, and often from punching a door.
21. **Never wear flip-flops** to run, walk your dog or climb a ladder.
22. **Power tools, tree stands, and ladders don't mix well with alcohol.**
23. **Same with anything fire-related**: Fireworks, fire pit, bonfire
24. **Take your meds as prescribed**. Your seizure meds, your blood pressure meds, your other meds. Except for other people's meds. Don't take other people's meds. Not even if they're the same color.

25. **Make good choices.** It's not funny, I know.

A previous version of this article was initially published 3 March 2019 on RadaJonesMD.com ©RadaJonesMD

THE PERFECT DOCTOR

I'm an ER doc. I spent my last two decades in the house of medicine. First, training to become a doctor. Then, trying to be a better doctor. But, no matter how hard I tried, I've never been close to being a perfect doctor. So I started wondering: what makes one a perfect doctor?

The perfect doctor lives in the moment, focusing on here and now: This patient. This case. This encounter. They devote their undivided attention and all their energy to being present in the moment, putting everything else aside for now – the lousy Press-Ganeys, being late to his kid's soccer game, their back hurting since they're working the seventh shift in a string of ten.

The perfect doctor is up-to-date. Since medicine is always changing, the perfect doctor learns every day. They know all about vaping, they're aware that kayexalate is a curse, not a treatment, and they're ready to prescribe Buprenorphine from the ED. As Dr. Stuart Swadron says: **They**

know everything they need to know, and a little more. They are curious, since there's so much that they don't know. We don't even know what we don't know. Curiosity opens the door to the miracles of the world.

The perfect doctor is often wrong, since being wrong allows you to learn. Those who are always right have nothing to learn.

The perfect ER doc is efficient and chooses wisely. They don't do three consecutive workups on the same patient while the waiting room overflows with sick people fixing to die. The perfect ER doc takes well-calculated risks.

They are humble. Once you understand that your success is largely due to your DNA, the circumstances of your birth, and your luck, you'll also understand that others are just as responsible for their failures as you are for your success. There but for the grace of God go I.

They are hard on their opinions. As the Australian comedian Tim Minchin said: "Opinions, like assholes, need to be examined regularly. Make sure yours are up to par."

They are kind. They know that anxiety, stress and PTSD can be more deadly than many lethal diseases, and they strive to provide hope and solace, even when they can't cure.

They listen. Sometimes people aren't there to listen, they're there to talk, and need to feel heard. The perfect doctor makes time to listen and speak to families, even when other patients are waiting to be seen, and grandma's only here for her worsening dementia. They know that, to her people, she's the one that matters.

They support, respect and nurture nurses. If

doctors are the officers in the war against death, nurses are the soldiers laying it all on the line. Nurses get bit, kicked and spat at. They have to deal with unkind patients, angry families and arrogant doctors, often on an empty stomach and a full bladder. They need and deserve gratitude, love, and support.

The perfect doctor treats grumpy consultants gingerly. Consultants are people too. Sleep deprivation and being chained to a pager won't make anyone a better person. And, for the good of your patient, sometimes it's not what you know, it's who you know.

The perfect doctor teaches, kindly. They teach patients, families, nurses, interns, students, colleagues. It's: You remember that…" as opposed to: "Don't you know that…"

They respect everybody equally, from the CEO to the janitor. We are not what we do. We are who we are and we all deserve respect.

The perfect doctor forgives. They forgive the spitting, the four-letters words, the patient who lied to them. Forgiving makes you a better human and a better doctor. It's hard to be a good doctor if you dislike your patients.

The perfect doctor has a sense of humor. They laugh at situations, at life, at themselves. Laughing is a language everybody understands, even babies and pets. Laughing brings people together. Laughing heals.

They cry. Hurting for your patients will make you a better doctor. As one of my mentors, Dr. Greg Henry said, "**Nobody cares how much you know, until they know how much you care.**"

They take care of themselves. A burned-out

doctor is not a good doctor, like a burned-out bulb is not a good bulb. To care well for others, you first need to care for yourself. You are your most valuable resource. Don't waste it.

The perfect doctor finds meaning in what they do, even when none is apparent. As Dr. Mel Herbert says: "**Remember that what you do matters.**"

They define themselves by what they love, not by what they hate. They focus on the good in people, on the great cases, on the lovely encounters. They bring a smile to people's faces.

The perfect doctor knows they aren't perfect. Nobody is, because perfection doesn't exist. Looking for perfection is like chasing the Holy Grail: It takes you far from what you love, and it never ends.

A previous version of this article was published 6 Dec 2019 on Doximity.com ©RadaJonesMD

MORE ER LAWS

1. **Pain's First Principle**: All patients with high pain tolerance are allergic to Motrin and Tylenol.
2. **Pain's Second Principle**: 95.8 percent of Fibromyalgia flares occur on Mondays.
3. **Pain's Rule of Furniture**: Chronic back pain patients live to move refrigerators.
4. **DeBeer's Law of Correlation:** The likelihood of a patient being suicidal correlates directly with the blood alcohol level.
5. **Fahrenheit's Law:** Parents of unvaccinated kids don't own thermometers.
6. **Poor's First Law**: Smoking is inversely correlated with the ability to afford your antibiotics.
7. **Poor's Second Law:** The number of tattoos is inversely correlated with being able to afford dental care.

8. **Poor's Corollary**: Beware the tooth to tattoo ratio.
9. **Hope's Law**: Being on Chantix negates smoking.
10. **Love's First Law**: The patient asking for your phone number is in the ER for an STD.
11. **Love's Second Law**: The patient who hugged you before he left has scabies.
12. **Love's Third Law:** The patient who shook your hand is positive for C-Diff.
13. **Pooper's Rule:** Patients with three weeks of diarrhea become constipated as soon as they step in the ER.
14. **Cheeto's Rule**: Abdominal pain gets better with Cheetos.
15. **Sucker's Law**: When you separate fighting dogs, you'll be the one who gets the shots.
16. **Amal Mattu's Law**: If the patient is so diaphoretic that you can't stick his EKG leads, just activate the Cath Lab. They're having a STEMI.
17. **L'Hospitel's Law**: Patients who need admission have pets at home they need to care for. **L'Hospitel's Reciprocal:** Patients who don't need admission have families that can no longer care for them.
18. **Tester's First Law**: Whenever you need a CTA, the patient's GFR is bad. **Tester's Reciprocal**: Whenever the GFR is bad, you need a CTA.
19. **Tester's Second Law:** D-dimers are positive only if the patient can't get a

CTA. **Tester's Corollary**: Then, they are positive every time, and the VQ scan is out of substrate.

20. **Luck's Theorems**: The likelihood of the computer crashing is directly proportional to the number of patients in the department. Multiply by five if it's Monday night. Add 10 if it's a full moon. If you're red-haired and have at least one stepparent, divide by 0.25.
21. **Schift's First Law**: JACHO only comes during *your shift.*
22. **Schift's Second Law**: The other doctor has fewer patients.
23. **Lavoisier's Principle on Medication Errors**: They always got too much. If they got too little, it would be easy to fix.
24. **Lavoisier's Theorem**: Tylenol allergy is a risk factor for fibromyalgia, IBS, and anxiety.
25. **Lavoisier's Rule of Anticoagulation**: Every patient who has a sloped porch must be on Coumadin.
26. **Lavoisier's Dictum**: When the patient comes to the ER, the med list stays home.
27. **Child's Principle**: Toddlers can't swallow pills. Unless they are grandma's. Then they'll swallow the whole bottle.
28. **Child's Law of Location**: Bleach can only be stored under the sink in a Coke bottle.
29. **Snow's Method**: The best way to unclog a snowblower is sticking your hand in it.
30. **Needy's First Rule:** Your patient will need you as soon as you leave the room.

31. **Needy's Second Rule**: Your consultant always needs the one test you didn't order.
32. **Margarita's Law**: The ER goes to shambles as soon as the pizza arrives. **Margarita's Corollary:** Never order pizza in the ED. **Margarita's Conclusion:** To eat hot pizza you need to retire.
33. **Bell's Rules**: Patients who are hard of hearing don't have their hearing aids. **Bell's first corollary**: If they do, the battery is dead. If it's not, the family will take them home, together with their watch, their jewelry, and their glasses
34. **Bell's Axiom**: If the patient doesn't speak English, the translation phone is not working. In the unlikely event that the phone is working, the patient will speak the only language that the phone does not.
35. **Sage's First Advice**: Skip the CT if the patient with abdominal pain is eating McDonald's.
36. **Sage's Second Advice**: Whenever a patient tells you: "You took care of my mom," don't ask how she is. She's dead.
37. **Sage's Third Advice**: The family member looking like the patient's mother is his wife. Don't ask.
38. **Sage's Unavoidable Error**: You should have called the other consultant first.
39. **Sage's Chest Pain Rule**: Every patient with chest pain, elevated troponin, and

cardiac risk factors has GERD. Just ask your cardiologist.

Initially published 15 Jan 2019 ©RadaJonesMD

DO YOU SPEAK ER?

You may not know it, but there's a language specific to emergency rooms. It's really not a language so much as… a common-sense collection of what to say and especially what not to say.

The things to say are easy: "Please." "Thank you." "I appreciate your care."

The things to never say? That's a little trickier. Here's a list of things that ER people hate to hear. I apologize if you find them offensive. We do too.

1. "Boy, it sure looks quiet here tonight."

In the ER, the "q-word" is "the one that shall not be uttered." Ever. Once uttered, the q-word will conjure the forces of darkness, and disaster will strike with the force of a full moon on Friday the 13th. I haven't yet killed anyone for saying the q-word, but rumor has it the ghosts of those who have died for saying it still haunt the ER.

2. "I have a high pain tolerance."

In ER lingo, that usually means: "I have a high

tolerance for pain medicines. Give me more." We won't. A variation on the theme is: "My pain is a 16 on a scale of one to 10." That's a no-no. In my 15 years in the ER, the two patients I've seen in the most horrific pain were both an eight. One had a small bowel obstruction. The other had an amputated leg—that arrived in a separate car. If your pain is 16 and you're texting while eating chips, you're out of luck. We don't do 16.

3. "98.9 is a fever for me."

No, it's not. You don't get to choose your own fever. You are human and therefore entitled to the same vitals as every other human—most mammals, in fact. You're allowed to call it a fever if you happen to be a leatherback sea turtle, whose core temperature is 78 degrees, or a crocodile, whose core temperature is around 91. But, if so, you should probably go see a vet.

4. "You have my allergies/medications/history in the computer. Go find them." Or: "Call my wife. She knows them." Or: "Call my doctor. The one at the office down the road from Ruby Tuesday. His name starts with a Z."

When you tell me to go look elsewhere for things you should know because you don't want to be bothered, I don't get the warm fuzzies. That's not cool. I have people dying to see me, so that leaves little time to call your wife about your meds. Arriving in the ER with a list of your meds, your known allergies, and the name of your doctor will make you very popular.

5. "Do I really have to tell you again? You're the third person asking me! Can't you just speak to each other?"

As a matter of fact, we do speak to each other, but we need to speak to you too. The fact that you told registration your chief complaint—in between giving them your insurance card and spelling out your middle name—does not provide me with an adequate history of your current medical situation. It's a whole lot easier for all of us if you help me help you.

6. "I've had this pain for two years. I've seen five specialists. I'm not going home without an answer."

You may be here for a long time, my friend. In case you were unaware, the "E" in ER stands for "emergency." We're unlikely to find an answer that five specialists took two years not to find, and we're likely to cost you, or your insurance, a lot of money.

7. "I have an allergy to Tylenol and Motrin, but Percocet works for me."

If Percocet works, you don't have an allergy to Tylenol. Percocet is 90 percent Tylenol—plus the good stuff. The good stuff doesn't cancel the Tylenol; it just makes it better.

8. "I have an appointment with my doctor in an hour, but I didn't feel well enough to see them." Or "I didn't want to wait."

Newsflash: Unless your doctor is a plastic surgeon specializing in Botox injections, their purpose is to care for sick people. The best time to see them is when you're not feeling well. When you are feeling well, you should go find better things to do.

9. "I was here before them. Why do they get to go first?"

This is the ER, not McDonald's. It's not first

come, first served. We triage, which means we see the sicker people first, no matter how long anyone's been waiting. If you're here for a work note and they need the Cath lab, you'll have to wait.

10. "No offense, but I don't like doctors."

That's your right, but what are you expecting me to do with that? How would you feel if I started our relationship by telling you: "No offense, but I really hate patients"? (For the record, I don't.)

11. "I have no medical problems."

Then you hand me the list of 17 meds you take every day.

12. "I don't believe in vaccines."

What are you here for? If you don't believe in one of the very few things the entire medical community agrees on, then I'm not sure how we can help you. You should probably go see Jenny McCarthy instead.

13. "I haven't been able to keep anything down since last January."

If so, you are a medical miracle, and you belong in a museum rather than my ER. People can live a month without food and a couple of days without water. If you've been doing it for 10 months, you should contact the Guinness book of records.

14. "I lost my Dilaudid prescription, but I still have the one for penicillin." Or: "I forgot them in Finland. "Or: "The dog ate my script."

Rejoice, my friend! You are not alone. Dogs seem to have a penchant for opiate prescriptions in particular. There's a dog conspiracy out there, trying to rid the world of narcotics overuse. Be grateful!

15. "I googled my symptoms. They said I could die! I need to be seen right now!"

Stay Away from MY ER and Other Fun Bit... 147

If it's not Google, it's Dr. Oz, or a cousin's brother-in-law who knows somebody who's a nurse. Newsflash: Regardless of what Dr. Oz, Dr. Google, or Dr. Pepper told you, you'll have to wait for your turn.

16. "If somebody doesn't come see me in 10 minutes, I'm leaving."

This is not really a threat to us - we'll survive either way. I wish we could say the same for you.

17. "Why do you work in the ER? Why not specialize in something?"

Believe it or not, ER is a specialty. We are as specialized as it gets. Others specialize in specific organs—brain, heart, kidney—or specific types of patients—pediatrics, geriatrics, oncology. We specialize in time. We are "the first 15 minutes" specialists. We're here to keep you alive, then send you home or hand you over to other specialists. That's what we do, and nobody does it better.

18. "My doctor sent me here to get an MRI."

No, they didn't. They sent you here so they could go home for dinner. If they needed you to have an MRI, they'd order it for you – or call us.

19. "Why am I here today? You're the doctor, you tell me!"

I don't know much about you, except that you can talk, but don't feel like telling me why you're here. Then you may be better off seeing a pediatrician or a vet, since they specialize in nonverbal patients.

20. "Can you hold a moment?"

Said with a lifted finger to silence me, and your eyes glued on the TV – or your phone. No, I can't. Normally, I'd be happy to sit and chill, but my patients won't let me. The little old lady with dangerously low blood pressure, the three people with chest pain, and the kid who can't breathe prefer that I keep moving. Sorry for disturbing you. I'll be back sometime.

Initially published 22 Nov 2018 ©Rada Jones MD

LESSONS FROM MY PATIENTS

Through my many years of doctoring, I must have seen thousands of patients, but I only remember a few. The ones that I really liked, the ones that I really didn't, and those who taught me and made me grow, making me the doctor I am today.

I was still a junior resident when I saw an elderly black man with a lump at the base of his neck. I didn't know what it was, and ultrasounding it didn't help. I spoke to my attending. "Whatever it is, it's an outpatient workup. Send him home," he said.

I had no choice. I sent him home without treatment or diagnosis. He didn't mind. He gave me a toothless smile and said:

"You really enjoy what you're doing, don't you?"

I did. I didn't think he would care or even notice. But he had. He wanted to see me again if he came back. There was no way, of course - in the ER, you see whoever's there. I never saw him again, but he taught me that people need you to care about them even more than caring for them. What mattered most to him was how much I enjoyed caring for him.

As my mentor, Dr. Greg Henry, said: **"People don't care how much you know until they know how much you care."**

I was a brand-new attending when I took care of a septic old lady who needed a central line. I struggled. By the time I got it, I had given her a pneumothorax. Then she needed a chest tube, and I was devastated. I was the worst doctor in the world. I didn't want to see another patient. Ever. My colleague saw me seething.

"What's wrong?"

I told him. He laughed.

"Did you get in the central line?"

"Yes."

"Did you get in the chest tube?"

"Yes."

"So, why are you so upset?"

"I caused her unnecessary pain and suffering. If I were a better doctor, she wouldn't have needed the chest tube."

"A pneumothorax is a well-known complication of central lines. If you never caused one, you didn't put in enough central lines."

That helped. I went to see my other patients. My patient eventually left the hospital alive. Fifteen years later, I still remember what our encounter taught me.

Mistakes happen, but you can't focus on them. Learn your lesson, then go back and care for your patients.

The next case I remember wasn't that long ago. The patient, a man in his 40's, was DOA- dead on arrival. He came in as a trauma code: "crushed by a refrigerator." We coded him for an hour without getting a pulse. By the time his wife and children arrived, we had stopped.

Four of his five kids waited outside. The wife came in with the oldest, an eight-year-old. She had been with her father when he opened the refrigerator door to get a beer, and collapsed, pulling the refrigerator over him.

They were alone. She tried to push the refrigerator away, but couldn't. It was too heavy. She ran to the neighbors for help, half a mile, barefoot in the snow. They called 911. The ambulance took her father. She waited home for her mother, then they all came to the ER.

The mother was distraught. She cried, she screamed, she cursed her dead husband. It was his fault: his smoking, his drinking, his lack of medical care.

The child listened, her wide eyes dry, glancing from her mother to her father. She was a tiny little thing with a low, greasy ponytail, and clothes that could do with some washing. She shouldn't have watched her father's death, nor her mother's pain, anger, and cursing. But she had, and I couldn't help it.

The one thing I could do was to recognize her heroic effort to save her father. I thanked her for what she had done. I told her that nobody could have saved her father. I didn't want her to feel guilty for the rest of her life, thinking that if she only managed to get that refrigerator off her father, he'd still be alive. Nobody could have done better — not even me.

Her mother heard. She turned to her daughter

and hugged her, and the child started to cry. I'll never forget this little girl and her mother.

Sometimes you can't help the patient. But you're there to help whoever is in pain, whoever suffers, whoever needs you.

A version of this article was initially published on Doximity.com,©RadaJonesMD

ABOUT THE AUTHOR

Rada Jones is an American physician and author. She was born in Transylvania, just miles away from Dracula's castle.

She earned a degree in mechanical engineering from the University of Brasov, an MBA from the University of Quebec in Montreal and a Doctor of Medicine from the University of Connecticut. She practiced Emergency Medicine in the US and on cruise ships all over the world, but she still speaks like Dracula's cousin.

She lives in the Adirondacks with her husband and a German shepherd named Guinness who stars in some of her books. If she's not on some trail, she's either reading or traveling to faraway places.

Find more of her writing at RadaJonesMD.com.

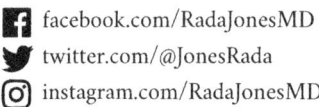

facebook.com/RadaJonesMD
twitter.com/@JonesRada
instagram.com/RadaJonesMD

OTHER BOOKS BY RADA JONES

ER CRIMES Series : What if the one supposed to save your life is trying to end it? Find out in *'ER Crimes,'* the chilling thriller series that will leave you breathless.

K-9 HEROES Series: "Until you, hoomans, learn to sniff each other's butts so you can read each other's thoughts, you'll need us, dogs, to guide you, love you, and make you better people.

THE CURSE OF THE DRACULA BROTHERS Series: Three magic spies. Two clashing empires. A deadly game no one survives.

DRIVING ITALY: Two intrepid curmudgeons. An SUV with red plates. Ten thousand miles of twisty roads. What could go wrong?

PRAISE FOR RADA JONES MD

As a retired ER doc, I like to post interesting articles for friends, nurses and doctors. I came across articles written by Rada Jones, MD. I was captivated by the insight, intelligence, humor, the sheer brilliance of her writing. Everything I wished I could come out with! I felt like I had come across the Mother Lode. I shared nuggets of gold with friends and colleagues. They loved her writing! What happened next was totally unexpected. One article got 38,000 shares, another 27,000. This was a testament to the brilliance of Rada's writing.

A few felt that some of the articles were offensive. I think that finding humor in the Catch-22 absurdities that we in the ER too often find ourselves in, is not only ethical, it is cathartic and therapeutic.

Katherine Watson from Northwestern University's Feinberg School of Medicine, a medical ethicist writes: "To me, the butt of the doctors' humor is not the patient. It's death. Not only did humor not harm anyone, but it helps doctors and nurses integrate this terrible event and get through the shift."

In so doing, the joke may help the next patient get the best possible care.

Rada Jones is a medical treasure. Enjoy.

Peter H. Chow MD

OVERDOSE: AN EXCERPT

Spider

"*He's not on.*"

They're lying. "*He told me to come back tonight. He said he'll be on after 3,*" I say, smiling like I like them.

Fuck them. Fuck them all.

"*He's not,*" says the fat one with the droopy mouth. She rechecks the papers.

"*No, not tonight. You've got it wrong.*"

I shrink under her gaze. I take out the package. I show it to her.

"*I got this for him.*"

The package is tired. I've been carrying it around. I got it squished under my arm so many times it's shaped like my armpit. It's still white-like, but the bow's about to fall off.

It looks secondhand. It is. I found it in a garbage bin. It smells it too, like smoke and booze and sweat.

Never mind, the knife inside it is sharp. I checked. I sliced through a tree branch with a flick of the wrist. It's an old hunting knife shaped like a fish, its scaly handle *growing into a long, smooth, solid blade thick enough to cut through ribs.*

I'm the hunter. I'm gonna get my kill.

Tonight or tomorrow, I'm gonna get him.

I make myself small. They like it when you're small. Makes them feel big and strong.

I bend my good right knee a bit more and slump my shoulders.

"Got it wrong then. Sorry. When's he on?"

She looks at me, her sharp eyes getting soft. I don't matter; I'm nothing to worry about. I'm small and old and dirty. She's sorry for me.

"I can't tell you," she says. "It's against the rules."

I rub my left eye, the one with the infection. It tears. "I just wanna thank him," I say. "He helped my son; he's a great doctor." *I look down and make myself smaller.* "I have a gift for him."

I show her the box again.

She breaks. She looks at the papers and says, "Tomorrow. Tomorrow at 9. He'll be here."

I rub my eye and thank her. I leave slowly, limping on the left like I always do.

I don't rush until I'm out in the dark and I know she can't see me. They can't see me.

Tomorrow at nine.

My knife and I, we have a date.

Made in the USA
Monee, IL
08 April 2024